A LAYMAN'S GUIDE
WHERE THE MIND IS IN THE BRAIN

A LAYMAN'S GUIDE
WHERE THE MIND IS IN THE BRAIN
AN EVOLUTIONARY AND ANATOMICAL PERSPECTIVE

MARIOUS KIM JACK, M.D.

Library of Congress Control Number: 2009904041
ISBN: Hardcover   978-1-4415-3157-5
          Softcover   978-1-4415-3156-8

This book was printed in the United States of America.

To order additional copies of this book, contact:
Xlibris Corporation
1-888-795-4274
www.Xlibris.com
Orders@Xlibris.com
58142

CONTENTS

PART III

How An Individual Human Recapitulates Human Evolution

DEDICATION

Over one hundred-fifty years ago biological science was put on notice by the inquisitive stirrings of Friedrich Zschokke, who proposed a bold and contrary theory regarding the physical state of the human mind. His assertion, a preposterous notion then and for most now, stated the mind was like the human brain in that it had evolved from a microscopically simple to a complex structure in the process of a progressive evolution which he labeled "the geology of the person". His unusual theory was likely inspired by Darwin and others who began to see animal behavior in humans. While Darwin is given the credit for Freudian inspirations about the mind, it is Zschokke who actually incited their incubation.

One of the most seminal investigators of modern enquiry regarding a brain with an evolutionary character was Paul D. MacLean, M.D., a professor at the Yale University School of Medicine and later director of the laboratory of Brain Evolution and Behavior at the National Institute of Mental Health. He investigated human behavior using animal brain models of experimentation. It is to him this book is dedicated.

MacLean's studies are now considered contrarian by some experts on the evolution of human cognition, especially Terrence Deacon, PH.D. of the University of California, Berkeley. His arguments to that effect claim that brain systems did not evolve by accretion; "instead the same brain structures have become modified in different ways in different lineages"*

Accretion by its definition, however, is the process of enlargement by gradual build up and easily applies to an evolutionary brain theory that reveals stages of increasing complexity. Deacon's position of opposition seems moot because in brain anatomy and animal behavior there is evidence of both accretion and modification of the earliest forms of animal nervous systems.

MacLean is of monumental importance to the understanding of the human condition even though his views have become unpopular because he has reined in the divergent accountability of the mind being explained one way and the brain another. In his voluminous works and his precision of scientific reasoning there began a subtle assertion that the evolved human "triune brain" has three "mentalities". With this seemingly oxymoronic synthesis, he gave science an invitation to treat mind and brain as one, not as separate. His insights compiled in his magnum opus,

---

* "A Theory Abandoned But Still Compelling" by Peter Farley, *Yale Medicine*. Autumn 2008, New Haven, Ct.

The Triune Brain in Evolution, documents human behavior outside the confines of the mind-brain dichotomy and makes a special point that much of man's behavior has genetic neurological origins.

The present text, *Where the Mind is in the Brain, a Layman's Guide*, is designed by the author to define with a simplified narrative the complex vernacular of MacLean's neuroscience. It is meant to be a primer of a very emotional subject that extends far beyond his scientific detractors. In addition, the author hopes to provide some additional insights about human behavior based on a layered triune mind-brain theory while reminding readers that both mind and brain with their evolutionary origins have two halves that must be successfully recapitulated in every newborn, otherwise there will be regressive behavior anomalies characteristic of previous stages of brain evolution.

PART I

A Brief Description of the Evolutionary
Events That Led to Human Self-Identity

PART I

Introduction

"Suppose you wanted to figure out how a radio would work. First thing you would do is make a parts list—take the radio apart and put all the component parts on the table. Then you'd figure out where they were. You have to understand how the interconnected parts in a biologic circuit work, and how they interact with other circuits in the cells."
Leroy Hood, President of the Institute for Systems Biology, Seattle, Washington

Evolution by its very definition tells us that in the biologic world there is a continuous line of derivation in which simple species give rise to more complex ones over distant epochs. This once unfathomable apostate proposition of organic transformation had its ancient origins in geological observations of Aristotle and Herodotus who first recorded the presence of fossilized shellfish in the western mountains that flank the Nile Valley. During the Middle Ages, shells and petrified fishes embedded in rocks aroused the curiosities of the Swabian Dominican friar, Albertus Magnus, and the Frenchman, Palissy. Yet it wasn't until the eighteenth century that Buffon of Burgundy laid the foundation for the concept of evolution with his observation of fossil types: "the less perfect species, those that were more delicate, heavier, less active or less well armed have already vanished or will vanish with time." Later, seizing upon this idea, Cuvier, Lamarck, Saint Hilarie and Darwin brought to scientific light the evolutionary concept that all species derived one from another, the more simple having given rise to the more complex.

Of contemporary interest is the appreciation of the mechanism of evolution and indeed, the object of this dissertation, are the observations of Teilhard de Chardin. He describes the progressive changes of the nervous systems of the various species during evolution: from simple cellular forms of protozoa to complex mammalian forms, by way of the

Coelenterata, Echinoderms and the lower vertebrates. In evolution, there is a greater organization of the nervous system of animals in which "the irreversible complexification and cephalization of the nervous system" has evolved. Delacato makes the argument by defining specifically the anatomy of the human nervous system as having increasingly complex components which by themselves can be identified as the complete nervous system of other animal species.*

In the late 1800rds, the Darwinian protagonist Ernst Heinrich Haeckel, a German biologist, not only substantiated the comprehension of a continuous evolution with observable microscopic evidence, but also posited a fundamental characteristic of its generic manifestations. First examining embryos of different mammals at a given time of their development, he identified that all mammalian species morphologically appeared the same but later matured into specific species. He further observed in human embryological development transformations that were characteristic of other more simple forms of life. At eight days, the fertilized ovum grows to a hollow sphere (blastula) similar to the morphology of sponges. The embryo then becomes a two-layered cuplike structure (gastrula) that is similar to coelenterates, the jellyfish and corals. Within thirty days, it passes through stages of development in which gills and tail and finlike limbs appear. From his observations, he proposed that "ontogenesis recapitulates phylogenesis" i.e. each animal in its individual embryological development from conception retraces the evolutionary steps of life from single celled organisms to more complex ones.

Haeckel's theory when applied to the maturation of the human nervous system reveals a biogenesis in which human neurologic components, characteristic of nervous systems of other species of animals, become more complex and integrated. In individual development there is a progression of neurological organization that proceeds vertically to the cortex of the human brain as myelinization takes place. This sequential progression is required to achieve the brain's fullest cerebral capability. Every human brain, to reach its greatest expression, must develop in a process of a linked recapitulation as Haeckel described it.

---

* The dogfish, rays and Chimaevas are the earliest form of vertebrates that have complete and separate vertebrae, movable jaws and paired appendages. Anatomically the brain of these animals primarily is controlled by the medulla. In the human, the medulla is only a component of an intricate brain. The reptile, a more complex vertebrate than the dogfish, has a large mid-brain as well as a medulla. In the human, the mid-brain along with the medulla, are just components of his more elaborate nervous system.

While the human has been thoroughly studied from this evolutionary prospective, the human mind, the consciousness that originates in the brain and directs mental and physical behavior has been exempt from an evolutionary analysis. The early appreciation of the mind as having an evolutionary character, first occurred to Haeckel who in 1899 proposed a *phylogenetic psychology* of the human thought process that paralleled the same evolutionary and developmental process of the human brain that he had previously described. It was this germinal idea that transfixed the attention of Freud and Jung and inspired much of the psychoanalytical dogma that followed. Yet the dogma has come to be criticized as not really being a science. The awareness of an evolutionary recapitulative development of the psyche could not be sustained on fragmentary evidence of myth, folklore, archetypes and analytical theories of the unconscious. Freudian theory and Jungian concepts were purged along with their obscure origins in Haeckel.

There also has been an ongoing resistance, not just theological, to studying the mind as a science. Other psychology disciplines using scientific experimentation with animals and humans have been challenged. They, too, have been the object of great debate and rejection because of what is critical to science, defining of elemental parts, identifying component parts and understanding how their interconnections work; what is understood to be reductionistic mechanics. Slobodkin, an evolutionary biologist proclaimed in the 1970's that man's mind cannot be understood by the laws applicable to other mammals even though their brains have a very similar physiology to ours. In 1980, Morowitz attacked the whole idea of human brain evolution in his *Rediscovering the Mind*. To him, the human mind, having consciousness, and having thoughts, could never be explained by reducing the mind to a biologic basis of enquiry. The scientific study of the mind by reductionism was considered by the psychologist, Gooch, as one of the major (scientific) disasters of our time. R. D. Laing puts the issue in terms of existential phenomenology wherein a subjective person exists contrary to a scientifically studied "organism". "If man is seen as an organism, therefore, there is no place for his desires, fears, hope, or despair." Thus reductionism, the process of explaining human behavior through comprehension of smaller functional units such as brain components and systems becomes a dangerous process. As Morowitz states: "If we envision our fellows solely as animals or machines, we drain our interactions of humanistic richness. Reductionism offers very little in the area of moral imperatives and removes moral responsibility for human actions."

Theoretical-scientific thinking about the mind has not been entirely abandoned in spite of contrary convictions. Contemporary scientific investigation of the mind is forging ahead with new theories and systems experimentation of how the mind works and how it evolved. The work of comparative and human anatomists, paleontologists, psychologists and neurologists are daring to invade the exclusionary solitude of the human mind with anatomical and evolutionary scrutiny and to think outside of the mind-brain box. In counter distinction to the opposition of evaluating the mind scientifically, it is the purpose of this book to unearth Haeckel's forgotten appreciation of the psyche's evolutionary character and its recapitulation in each newborn human being. Morality need not be swept away while we study and verify scientifically what the mind is. While the mind may not turn out to be just an evolutionary brain mechanism, there is too much to lose by taking a "hands off" position of attempting to understand how the mind works from the perspective of a physical science. Even if the mind is materialized from a subjective state to an objective component of the brain, reduced to an anatomical evolutionary scientific reality, the process holds no patent solution to life's eternal mystery.

Chapter 1

THE LAND OF OZ

HOW THE FIRST CELLULAR SELVES BECAME CO-DEPENDENT
WITH LARGER ORGANISMS.

At age seven, we know that girls and boys are intrigued with play which emulates adult behavior. Girls, grasping the art of motherhood, fantasize intently with dolls and dollhouses, while boys get vigorously fixated on toy soldiers in miniature games of combat. The virtual wars are not the silent movie kind, but accompanied by action sounds of boom, a rat-tat-tat, pawooh and other vocal assistance to the deployment of troops and destruction of the enemy.

Clarmont David Kaminski named by his parents in a reverence to some hoped for uniqueness, at the time of his interest in fanciful war, had no siblings and a parental attitude that frowned upon too much child indulgence. These circumstances provided him with plenty of time to devote to the microcosmic world of toy soldiers. Clarmont daydreamed to frightening extremes in his parents' eyes. Something had to be done. With some prodding accompanied by pouting, Clarmont was introduced into the company of another boy in hope some socializing would dampen his shyness.

The new playmate was Artimedus Onstine who fortunately liked the introverted life of the unreal as much as his new acquaintance. So much so, later in life, he spent most of his time with his nose in a book. Rather than submitting to head bashing by brutes on playing fields, he preferred to stay on the sidelines occupying himself with intellectual pursuits of Chinese cultures, the physical laws and the geologic record.

During the boys pre-pubescence however, they happily focused on their minds' imagined interests.

Their toy soldiers had World War I helmets which the British persisted in keeping during the Second Great War. The cadre consisted of marching men shouldering field rifles; others were firing 45 caliber hand guns and still others were lying prone or kneeling with their weapons aimed with a child's unerring accuracy at the bull's eye. The toy army had nurses, machine gunners and artillery with caissons to match. Lines of toy barbed wire were drawn between the good guys and the bad. Much of the enemy army had to be imagined, because collections of toy soldiers didn't include an over-whelming number of enemy forces. The boys seemed to have an uncanny sense of what Marshal Foch wrote in *The Principles of War*. There was a front line in a broad perimeter laid out on the living room rug; there were scouts in advanced positions, runners coming and going back to a secondary line of defense, and further back a central command headquarters where reserves and mechanized units were kept in the ready. With arms and hands moving soldiers at speeds that hid their animator's involvement, the make-believe world was spinning in its own reality. One day Artimedus got bored. There, before them, was the battle scene divided by a blue half-inch wide ribbon from Mrs. Kaminski's sewing basket. The ribbon was the Muse River; it was easy to see. All in array, the casualties lay strung on their backs and fronts slightly encumbered in those positions because of the metal platforms toy soldiers need. Artimedus rolled back on his knees, puffed up his lips allowing his cheeks to swell without the aid of bubble gum. He placed his hands behind his head in great deliberation about his disinterest of what now had become child's play.

Kaminski's face dropped in disappointment; he had hoped this sport would never end. He waited for his erudite buddy to begin his deliberation. "Let's pretend," as was always the case, "that this war is going on and a giant space rocket comes down and lands on top of the battle field and all these guys are trapped inside. We'll be the spacemen and we will talk to the generals and let them know how stupid they are. We're taking them back to another planet."

These young boys, isolated in the cocoon of their imaginations, had just enacted an early significant event in the evolution of human life. They were unknowingly playing a game about the human micro-immune system, the most elemental aspect of human self-identity.

Long before Precambrian times, at the beginning of life itself, single-celled animals were all there was to life in the seas and oceans. Those cells that are measured in microns, a measurement that is a one thousandth part of a millimeter, had a *self-identity* even though they were so small. They possessed a microscopic sense of self.

The term *self-identity* refers to the *complex characteristics by which organisms recognize themselves as separate from their environment.* All forms of life must have self-identity or they are just part of the endless cosmos. Without a self-identity they have no individual existence. The outer membrane of a single-celled animal is the border between life and death, self and non-self. These early single-celled animals have a lineage that has survived intact to this day. They are known as amoebas.

The primordial ancestors of the amoebas were frequently destroyed by too much heat, too much light, too much sound, the wrong PH as well as other kinds of excessive forces. They had a difficult time maintaining their self-identity. In order to do so, they had to eat, and like their kin today, they wandered about in aqueous environments and let food into their inner-selves through the cell membrane by means of a primitive ingestion called phagocytosis. Often their food was a flagellate predator or a sub-cellular organism which was later identified as a bacterium or a virus. After millions of years, those ancient amoebic cells became the first cellular element of the human micro-immune system.

As immunologists seek solutions for problems of immunity, they have not forgotten everything about living creatures. These scientists appreciate that the human immune system has had a long evolution. For instance, immunity is a reflection of an evolutionary process in which amebocytes once were ingested by coelenterates, but instead of being absorbed, they developed a symbiotic relationship with their hosts and became the first protectors of these more complex organisms. The amoebas were the rudimentary immune cells in the guts of the coelenterates. (Likewise, our immunity is not an assembly line package of human biologic protection that is instantly available to guard against microscopic cellular invaders. This micro-cellular immunity must develop as an essential building block of human self-identity.)

Shortly after the union of amoebic-like cells and their hosts, evolution also provided the "new" coelenterates with a specialized self-identity cell. With the evolution of increased numbers of cells doing specialized things for organisms, the specialized cells lost a great deal of their individual self-identity and it was entrusted not just to amebocytes but to a new identity cell, the nerve cell. The nerve cell would protect those many self-identity deprived cells of an organism from bigger predators and physical elements of destruction. The multi-cellular organisms now had two basic cell types to recognize where the self began and where it ended. The nerve cells would evolve to become the autonomic nervous system of the human body. Nerve cells would provide self-identity for both the inner and outer layers of cells of early organisms. Much later in evolution, all of man's inner organs would have their identity maintained by these nerve cells. The amebocytes would remain in their original job, but eventually would be controlled by the autonomic nerve cells. Something we now call a system of self-identity.

Over many millions of years, nerve cells evolved further to produce tiny brains in micro-animals, the first of which were the platyhelminths, the flat worms, and also very early on in evolution the clams. This development was the first evidence of an organ within an organism that had the specific function of providing self-identity. This rudimentary brain was primarily concerned with maintaining the survival of the organism. The brain's territory within which *self* was maintained, was not just the gut patrolled by the amebocytes, but also the limits of the organism's outer body.

Self-identity took its time. Through more millions of years, it remained limited to the body of primitive organisms. The body self was first identified from within, by the immune cells and nerve ending, and from without, by other nerve cell endings on the surface. These two types of cells protected against predatory organisms and injurious agents that got into the body through the gut and from predators attacking the body's surface. The *self* of animals had changed from being defined by a cell membrane to the surface dimensions of its inner and outer body defined by nerve cells and amebocytes.

Not abruptly, but from the beginning of single cell life, in slow increments of evolution, those early brains acquired sense organs that could pick up information short distances away from the perimeters of their bodies. As organisms evolved with backbones from fishes to amphibians, a subtle transition in the brains of those animals with new sensory organs occurred. They began to extend what they considered *self* to include things beyond the body, things that were in a watery space. These sense organs expanded survival by producing two fundamental functions. In evolution, cells that became organisms began to be concerned about what was out there away from the limits of their bodies. They asked. "Is the something out there to consume and sustain me, or something from which to escape?" The self-identity of the reptile's brain best defines that monumental change.

Chapter 2

THE REPTILE EXPANDS
ITS SENSE OF SELF

HOW ANCIENT REPTILES EVOLVED TO BE MORE THAN THEIR BODIES.

When David Kaminski was thirteen years old, he had no idea about gonadotropins and leutinizing hormones. He only appreciated that something unusual was happening to his body. Up to this time in his life, he was an undifferentiated chore person, raking lawns, cutting grass, taking out the garbage. But there appeared overnight a slight timbre to his voice and thread-thin velvety suggestions of a beard first above the upper lip and then in a tiny spot on his chin. Down below his navel more hair appeared; the texture was surprisingly different.

These body signs appropriately matched hidden urges that he hoped could be materialized in his new flesh. The first steps of involvement with the opposite sex had little to do with those corporal urges but more with a process that required a brotherhood action of those similarly maturing. Initially, there was no one-on-one confrontation. It was stalking within the comfort of groups of males gawking together in twos and threes. Just before the Second World War, there was a proper place that rivaled the "paseo" of ancient Hispanic wooing. In those by-gone days of the forties, the action took place at mixers in the hall of the Knights of Columbus where second-hand Stan Kenton, Tex Bennike and Tommy Dorsey made their auditory presence on big black discs within a Wurlitzer jukebox.

Getting out of the house on Friday night for Kaminski was an improvisation of indifference. "Gosh, there's nothing else to do," yawn. "Guess Robert Fitzsimmons and I'll go to a movie. See ya, Mom, I won't be late." Taking a quick look in the hallway mirror at his new maturity, he checked to make sure his fly was closed. Proceeding slowly with feigned boredom, once outside the door, his composure turned into a foot race so as not to be denied entry to a dance hall with a ticket, rubber stamped on his hand with ink that glowed in the dark. Kaminski and his pal, Fitzsimmons, left the evening's darkness only to enter into another. The illumination of the hall came only from the turntable. Humans were visible in the form of a merry-go-round of mostly female heads keeping time to the music. It seemed like half the night would pass before a few callow adolescent males overcame their gawky inhibitions. Finally, the nerve came to place a finger on the shoulders of female traffic in the outer orbit of a musical centrifuge. Two boys would "break in" as it was called, and now the two pairs of opposite sex would go round and round for the duration of a song that seemed to last only long enough to move a chin onto a forehead. When the music abruptly ended, it called for an expression of superhuman teenage male courage; "Can we dance the next one?"

Kaminski and Fitzsimmons, not even sure they would take the initial fatal step of breaking in, spotted an even more primal scene among the silhouettes of heads and shoulders. A junior from their high school was doing his second dance with a pretty young girl in a pleated skirt and bobby socks. She was from a high school in another part of town. Toward the main entrance of the ballroom, glowering at her, there appeared to be an older man but actually only nineteen years old. He was out of uniform for a dance in his blue US Navy seaman's outfit. It appeared his presence had nothing to do with dancing. He nervously brandished a silver bracelet with his name and an anchor on one side. His cronies, with eyes flickering and heads in feudal subservience, were waiting for sadistic rewards of impending battle.

This rogue sailor, home on leave, was reestablishing his territory and a relationship with a girl he left behind because he had flunked out of school. Boom went the gong in his prehistoric head. He strode forth making a beeline for his prey. His pumped-up physique of a middleweight was about to start the first round. That was what he loved to do most, boxing for prizes at his San Diego Naval Base. Moving couples aside with just his presence, he tapped Kaminski's acquaintance on the shoulder with a staccato of movement that demanded instant reply.

"Sorry, but we're still dancing." Another penetrating tap, and another, without the desired result.

"I'll see you outside, you little asshole."

The music stopped and sixty people rushed outside to a dimly lit alley. Grown men appeared and held out their arms to keep the teenage onlookers from crowding in. They were to referee in this trumped up survival of the fittest. Then the sailor began his onslaught with professional left jabs and right slams to the body. Out came bullet-speed triceps action to the jaw, over, and over again. Blood flowed from the amateur combatant's nose, from the corners of his bruised mouth. He fell to his knees. The jabs continued, followed by sustained and powerful punches. The victim's head rolled back. Boys and girls encircled two deep were taking it all in and getting edgy. Feeling powerless, they were intimidated by the adult bosses of the ring and the physical mayhem. Nobody intervened. It went on almost to unconsciousness until finally a cop stepped forward and rescued the kid, picked him up from the street now spotted with violaceous blood shining in the night.

Massaging his skinny biceps, a sickened Kaminski, knew how he would have fared.

The creatures that evolved after the coelenterates first had no spines, but later animals developed them during a period of almost three hundred million years. (It is necessary to take "photo stills" of that evolutionary process which occurred so slowly and imperceptibly. Similarly, we must turn our backs, from time to time, to appreciate that the moon is actually rising.)

The ancient reptile evolving out of all those creatures before him, was the most representative of the animals whose brains dramatically changed the character of future animal self-identity. In the beginning, this reptile confined to water, came out to dominate the land during the hundred million year period known as the Mesozoic era. (A survivor of those ancient reptiles today is the Komodo dragon.) The ancient reptile along with other vertebrates evolved with certain special nerve cells that developed specific sensitivities for specific kinds of energy. Light, heat, sound, vibration and smell sensory organs evolved out of their brains. (However, sense organs, especially for light, can be traced in their development throughout evolution from one-celled animals all the way up to the reptiles. The marker of development of an organ sense will be credited to the reptile.) These sense organs provided their owners with the ability to recognize combinations of special kinds of energy emitted by species-specific prey, mates, rivals, and predators. The initial recognition was limited and these reptiles treated all other creatures about the same, as a violent threat. The new sensory nerve cells attached to these special organs eventually acquired a new memory in the reptile's brain. They provided the animal the ability to recognize those specific animal objects of predation in the environment away from the reptile's body. The nerve cells evolved so that the reptile could sense the whereabouts of prey without stepping on it. These reptiles could sense the presence of predators before they came into physical contact with their own bodies. They did not need to be half-full of prey or half-eaten by predators before they knew what was happening. They could tell things were going to happen before they happened. Urges to fight or flight could take place at a distance.

These evolved reptiles did not need to experience actual body pain to survive. These reptiles had developed special sensory areas of their small brains that could anticipate pain. One self-identity nerve cell, however, stayed where it had originally evolved, under the skin of the animal, at the old junction between the body-self and the non-self. These body pain sensing identity nerve cells were minding the store as in the old days. They continued to tell the animal he was or wasn't at the border of his skin. These first identity nerve cells continued to allow the reptile, if bitten by a predator, to know the location and the moment pain was beginning. These first nerve cells also continued to cause pain in the animal's stomach that drove him to prey.

The first raw pain occurring on the skin of an animal was the sensation of actual tissue destruction, the end of self. With these new nerve cells of the special senses, pain could be appreciated before it occurred. These new special senses brought into being a simple, yet more advanced consciousness for the reptile. As always, he could experience raw pain if tissue destruction occurred, and with his new special senses he could *anticipate* pain. Anticipated pain could be appreciated with a consciousness of fear and anger. Reptiles could respond with fight or flight well ahead of tissue destruction.

These new sensory organs of the reptile's brain gave the reptile a greater chance of survival over invertebrates and other animals without them. They also put time and space between reptile bodies and early forms of energy that could cause tissue destruction. These new sense organs extended self-identity from the surface of the animal body to a territory that the reptile defended as if it were his body. No large animal was safe, no female, no rival, no predator, no offspring. The evolved reptile sense of self extended beyond its body limits to a territory defined by its special senses. The most important sense for the reptile to manage the territory was the sense of taste emanating from a forked tongue. His other senses took a back seat in his identification of reality.

Reptiles that have survived today, the Komodo dragons, the crocodiles and alligators have just a few things on their minds. They are conscious of actual pain inflicted by predators, rivals and mates and prey not yet in their stomachs. They are also conscious of fear and anger as a prelude to the action of fight or flight.

According to contemporary observations of reptiles, in addition to operating in a strict territory, they create and maintain rigid hierarchies among themselves for control of that territory. A dominance system among members of the same species evolved out of the sense of territorial self. (It is this ancient brain wiring that the human has also acquired. It is the brain structure that drives man's behavior as well.)

Reptiles and the mammals that evolved after the land based reptiles display stereotypical territorial and hierarchical behavior based on millions of years of ancestral learning. Reptilian behavior is essentially non-adaptive, not able to be modified through learning experiences during an individual reptile's life. A good example of the reptilian brain at work is found within the great sea mammal, the whale. Century after century, the whale comes back to specific breeding grounds where whalers lie in wait to destroy them. Comparative anatomy studies of mammalian brains demonstrate they have a reptilian component in their brains. What has been ascribed specifically to mammalian behavior actually is a product of their reptilian ancestry. (The reptilian component of the fur seal's brain provided the same inability to adapt as sealers decimated their numbers in the thousands.) No learning takes place, from year to year, about the danger of the breeding place; the whale and the seals have only learned they must come back. The hierarchical character of reptilian behavior is eloquently described by Konrad Lorenz in the brutal competitive behavior of rats toward members of their own species due to crowding which disrupts their social order. MacLean describes the will to power of two male rainbow lizards striving for dominance. "Like a return to the days of King Arthur these animals have beautiful colors and like many lizards, use head-bobbing and pushups in territorial and courtship displays. In a contest, once the gauntlet is throw down, the aggressive displays give way to violent combat and the struggle is unrelenting." There are some thoughts that the first kind of reptile, the dinosaurs, became extinct because their aggressive self-identity only barely relaxed during the actual act of mating. Even though reptilian courtship ends in copulation, it essentially is a process of combat between male and female, an aggressive conquering act of submission.

The old reptiles lacked a fundamental expansion of self-identity to include mates beyond a momentary mating and, as well, did not include offspring. Those dinosaurs were unable to protect their eggs during incubation. The eggs were gobbled up by other reptiles and eventually mammals. (What we see today, are surviving reptiles that have evolved to protect their eggs during incubation.)

Now, at this point in evolution, self-identity in animals has extended from the boundary of a body comprised of cells, to a territory and a "kill or be killed" hierarchical control of a den, rivals, food, mates and enemies. The reptile was not just his body anymore, through his bigger brain and his new senses he defended his territory by controlling all animals in that territory. In his brain, there was one catch; the moment the reptile did not have the smell, sight, sound, or primarily, the taste of those animals that challenged his self-identity, his sense of self had no conscious awareness. He would remain asleep until consciousness of pain from an empty stomach drove his body relentlessly to search his territory for prey. The new special senses had developed memory, but the memory was only for fleeting stimuli, on-going, actually present events impinging on his sensory receptors. There was no memory of things past or in a future beyond the immediate impressions of those primitive sense organs. When asked where he had put his new meal, the old reptile could not remember unless he could taste it in the air.

Chapter 3

OLD MAMMAL CHANGES IN THE REPTILIAN SENSE OF SELF

HOW EARLY MAMMALS EVOLVED TO HAVE A SELF-IDENTITY BEYOND A FIXED TERRITORY AND ONE THAT INCLUDED OTHER ANIMALS OF THE SAME SPECIES.

David Kaminski's father, Calvin, always looked forward to getting out of his provincial western town and traveling to New York City. He went there to participate in corporate conventions of the electrical industry that rallied around the emblem of Reddy Kilowatt. Kaminski's father would reap the benefits of travel provided by corporate life in the form of a per diem, in his day, simply called an expense account. By eating at automats, he often insured some money came home as surplus. Less tangible perks included relief from the grind of a corporate office not chalked up to vacation time.

There were new experiences only great cities like Manhattan or Chicago could offer. He would savor baklava and steak tartar, mingle on the crowded streets with ethnic types whose dark visages reminded him of his own. He would pay his first dollar tip to a cab driver and see real "bumps and grinds". In 1940, New York City was the Mecca for western executives to feel sophisticated, by whooping it up in hotels and clubs that catered to the likes of Walter Winchell. The corporate men, feeling no slight, were given tables in the back of clubs and dining rooms that thrived on an unsuspected caste system. To eastern corporate executives, western types were considered cowpoke celebrities themselves. They got that respect, because western power and electric corporations were listed on the New York Stock Exchange and always paid a handsome dividend. Westerners derived their own sense of importance when they traveled cross-country, the posh way, in a United Airlines sleeper coach.

An ex-Mormon, but unable to ever forget the disciplines required to be one, David Kaminski's father had to mix socially with the corporate in-bunch. Being one of the guys required behavior that was in conflict with his early teaching. Unfortunately, merits for promotion included participating in administrative duties that involved whiskey and cigars. Calvin Kaminski was going to be falsely true to both new demands and old convictions.

One hot summer day, while wading in hob-nail boots in the Pend Oreille River of Idaho's panhandle, he explained to his son how he did it. David Kaminski and his father were casting grey hackle dry-flies for cut throat trout in a deep, sap-green hole along the river's bank. Out of his wicker fish-basket, the company executive drew a pint-sized flask covered with tanned leather. With its chromed cap, it seemed more appropriate for a heavy drinking member of an African safari. It had been lying in his creel alongside thick blades of river grass that insulated the bodies of his catch. "You take a swig of booze just like this, son." He was referring to times in his hotel room where company men were letting off steam with Old Crow and Jack Daniel's whiskey. They would pass the bottle round and round, sanitized with the brush of a sleeve on the bottle's mouth. Staying sober was a form of corporate competition, and the CEO, president and chairman of the board, all in one man, watched his rivals and would-be heirs closely to see who could talk business and remain sober. The CEO would remember when bonuses and promotions were handed out, whose heads would remain erect above unwound ties and unbuttoned white shirt collars.

David Kaminski's father demonstrated his sly way of staying competitive for his boss's favors. With the cap off, after the sleeve sterilization, the pint went up to his mouth and addressed the face of the sky in the attitude of a bugler playing taps. Then David, the only observer, could see bubbles bouncing throughout the liquid-free, visible end of the bottle; gulps and swallows were simulated in believable earnest.

"You see, I haven't drunk a drop. I can out-drink any man this way, and I advise you to do the same or get thrown in jail for drunkenness.

David Kaminski, at fifteen years of age, would heed and emulate his father in many ways, especially his need to leave the home territory. The family car, a green 1938 Plymouth, stood in the driveway like a siren of the deep. Its attraction became as great as all the other things that appeal to that age. It came out of some unconscious desire that had no explanation. It was the means to an end—the open road. By clever study and experiment, the motor of the Plymouth was started and revved. The clutch pedal was exercised with grinding and then jerky movement. Eventually, tires turned back and forth along the driveway until the day the auto was driven with white-knuckled assistance of parents to the local department of motor vehicle licenses. Thereafter, for many summers, a voyage of exploration blinded David to any other interest. He was not alone. Some teenagers would take to hopping railroad cars of the Northern Pacific; others worked in pea fields to save money for the model "T" and still others had to face the impossible of borrowing the family car. There was a compulsive desire in young men's bones for movement out of the neighborhoods. They had to follow their ancestors' footsteps and see what was on the other side of the mountains.

The anthropologist Romer tells us that in the process of evolution, the brains of old mammals "enlarged enormously" about the same time they gave up producing eggs as a way of giving birth to the young. Most of this enlargement occurred in the new brain of old mammals called the *limbic brain*. It became also known as the *rhinencephalon*. (Very early evolving mammals persist today as the duck billed platypus of Australia and the spiny anteater of New Guinea. These mammals lay eggs and have many other attributes of reptiles.) But old mammals evolved further to produce their young by mechanisms with which we are all familiar. Along with a change in reproductive activities, some old mammals evolved to have fangs and claws which were ideal for flesh eaters, while other old mammals developed hooves and grinding teeth which were necessary for a vegetarian diet. Both kinds of old mammals broke the code of the reptilian sense of self; they changed the reptile's absolute control of a territory and the attacks on those in it.

The sense of self, an organism's self-identity, has an evolutionary character in which nothing is thrown away, only modified. There are no balls of torn up paper on the floor underneath the genetic typewriter with one, new, finished document. Instead there is one continuous roll of tissue paper production that spans over a billion years. In old mammals, "the sense of self" organ, the brain, contains a component which represents the smaller and less evolved brain of reptiles. Just as humans have a brain that also contains the components of brains of less-evolved animals. (The human brain became bigger as new, more complex brain parts were added to old ones.) There are new models off the assembly line, but these models still have parts of the prototype to which new parts are added, not substituted. It is as if you have two transmissions in one car and you have to use a stick shift with a clutch before you can use an automatic shift without the clutch.

Mammals changed their self-identity in new ground-breaking ways from the reptile, but the reptile could still be easily recognized in mammalian self-identity. Old mammals developed a self-identity that was not just defined by their own bodies and a fixed territory. Old mammals took the reptilian idea of self and added on a new part that modified it. Evolution of old mammals provided distinct changes from the reptile's only understanding of war against anything that came into its territory. Old mammals started to consider certain animals of their own kind as if they were themselves, just as small aquatic animals and the amebocytes did millions of years earlier. In a continuing process of evolution, the self-identity of old mammals was slowly incorporating more territory and more of their kind of animal as self. Old mammals extended their self-identity beyond a small territory to include mates, offspring, and some older rivals as if they were themselves. Self was extended to include more than a fixed territory and old mammals extended further to include offspring, while they grew up, and to mates, while the young were growing up. The sense of self also included older rivals especially while hunting prey and protecting their young. The chief males still kept hierarchical control of rivals, but not so absolutely, not so monolithically as the reptiles. Old mammal rivals would still fight to gain control of mates, dens, food and prey, but their newly evolving brains started to inhibit certain reptilian behavior. They stopped playing an absolute game of king of the mountain. Often two or more males would share leadership and dominate the hierarchy. They would share even the females and share care of offspring until the small fry rose to maturity. The old mammals began to share the territory and everything in it to a limited extent. They began hunting prey in cooperative teams. They defended the territory not one on one but as units. The first mammals developed a new way to handle internecine disputes regarding mating and maintaining their hierarchies. Their brains developed non-lethal, not so injurious displays of power and dominance. With vocal expressions of growls, visual expressions of baring teeth and more involved body postures, these early mammals could keep predators and rivals at a distance without engaging in reptilian combat. They learned to leave a uriniferous scent to mark the territory and could protect it without being present. These new behaviors could elicit fear and anger in rivals and mates without actually having to engage in lethal body combat. They increased the brain process of intimidation beyond the fleeting displays of reptiles.

Old mammals also broke out of the self-identity of reptiles regarding a fixed territory. They began to migrate beyond the territory. With an expanded area, these mammals could survive more readily because migration allowed them to go to new water holes, new grasslands and new prey. They could leave when predators became too numerous in the fixed territory. They were evolving a greater memory for areas that include places far away from what once was considered home. (The ungulates were not so intelligent with respect to hunting, of course, because they stayed with their vegetarian way of life, but their sharing and expansion of the territory became astronomical.)

From this evolved old mammalian brain that became incorporated into the human brain component, came the behavior of play and amicability in a family. (You could say love started here as you watch contemporary lions mate for hours.) The brain of old mammals created an inseparable neurological bonding that sustained itself for fixed periods between mother and child and male and female. it would bring to the human, emotions of abandonment, selflessness, the feeling of loneliness. It created a comfortable sense of being with a mate beyond the compulsion to copulate and flee.

Chapter 4

PRIMATE MANAGEMENT OF OLD MAMMALIAN MECHANISMS OF SELF

HOW PRIMATE MAMMALS LIVING IN TREES NEEDED A NEW FORM OF COMMUNICATION.

David Kaminski kissed his mother goodbye. Having just become aware of the incestuous taboo of lips to lips, he aimed at her cheek. Still reverent to his maternal dependence he accepted a token of its lesser status in the form of a brown bag that replaced a tin square lunch bucket with Disney designs. The bag would swing nicely from the same hand that carried both a notebook and a textbook with its own brown paper cover. In the bag, neatly wrapped in wax paper, was a tuna sandwich mixed with mayonnaise and sweet pickle. An orange adjoined the main course. Mrs. Kaminski looked longingly out of one of the entry parlor's side windows. With a faint-hearted smile she accepted with resignation that this was a special farewell. She knew this was the end of her little boy. Dressed in a tan windbreaker, white Arrow shirt, white corduroys, shoes with real leather heels, David began high school by assuming the fashion of high school juniors and seniors. At thirteen, he was about to begin four years of both formal and informal preparatory education. He would start a transformation of himself with experiences he hadn't yet dreamed. He entered into a new phase of life that bypassed the giving over of pubescent males by their mothers in a primitive ceremony demanded by their fathers. The process out of mothers' dens into the long houses of the males, was not to be accompanied by circumcision, the knocking out of two front teeth or having scars beautified with ashes from a campfire. His only physical token of passage was his braces that dully reflected light from any natural or artificial source of illumination.

This high school society he was entering, barred parents, teachers, clergy and anyone over eighteen years of age even though these aliens often intruded with their physical presence. This was a feudal, tribal, clannish society. It also had a Magdalenian stone age character, but most of all, it was a primate society.

The identities of members of the society were mostly appreciated visually. Freshmen were noted not to shave but on rare occasions. Their necks were skinny along with legs and arms that hadn't acquired the full effect of testosterone. They often breathed through their mouths due to childhood allergies. They also could be identified because they still carried white handkerchiefs in their pockets. They had no societal rights or position. They were the thralls hoping not to anger the lords. They stayed out of sight by not wearing their own glasses. For them, the opposite sex appeared only in the consciousness of wet dreams. We are talking boys here; for girls, it was a different thing. Ninth grade girls were like a new vintage wine, fresh and in no need of ripening.

The warriors, wearing athletic letter sweaters, were impossible to miss in their daily hallway parade. The royal dames of the upper classmen wore tight sweaters intended not to obscure their own two emblems of distinction. Those that had acquired noble status included the courtly that were considered by royalty to be popular, something Merlin would have had a hard time explaining. Then there appeared the kings and queens whose coronation had taken place on a parlor couch or a car's bench seat. Once attaining this nobility, these couples claimed the esteemed position of "going steady". The jewels in their crowns were the exchanged school rings or pins. Down the social order were members of the band, also those into the drugs available then, cigarettes and beer. Mixed unobtrusively with the freshmen were those that seemed to be without a real portfolio; they had come to high school unaware of its society only of its purpose to provide an education.

Kaminski didn't take long to size up his station in this new life. He could see that you had to be a class officer, work the special interest groups, or join the warrior class; what your mom and dad thought of you was of little concern. At first, it was a matter of survival not to be noticed as anything special, to be like all the other guys. Kaminski had his father's suppressive reticence so it was easy to be unobtrusive, to be overlooked and to appear withdrawn. What drove students to study was some vague remnant of parental supervision. To be thought of as intelligent was considered irrelevant until the day of graduation. For Kaminski, there was no wardrobe for his emerging libido, but it was kept under wraps with stolen darts of enquiry at legs of maturing females. While sitting in their classroom seats, he would drop a graphite pencil and retrieve it after it was propelled to come to rest at their feet. Using only his peripheral vision, he developed tension headaches trying to appear indifferent as he appreciated the great variety of nubile breasts. In four years, in spite of all the demands, Kaminski made his mark in that society, but to no avail, the assimilation and excitement of that world came to an end before he was ready to leave it.

The evolution of primates continued to change self-identity of reptiles beyond the modifications that have come to be identified with old mammals. Primates are well appreciated to be tree dwellers, but their brains evolved out of ground dependent old mammal brains and the behaviors that came from those brains. Old mammals utilized all of their special sense organs, eyes, ears, nose, tongue and footpads, but relied upon the sense of smell to best identify self from non-self. It would not be so for primates. Arboreal life had a profound effect upon which sense organs would evolve. Vision came to be more important for survival than any other of the major senses. The sense of smell failed to provide a satisfactory maintenance of life in the trees. While the sense of smell drove old mammals to prey and away from predators on the ground, it was a poor guide in performing those functions while swinging from tree to tree.

In the vision of primates, the images in the brain from the two eyes became overlapped and created stereoscopic images. A "central pit" developed in the retinas and the details of ticks and mites on the body and the accurate seeing of tree top rivals and predators became possible. On the motor side of the primate's brain that responded to acute visual stimulation, acrobatic body functions developed. A tail began to perform more duties for the body, and a hand with a thumb evolved out of footpads. Sitting upright, the primates with new grasping appendages could perform more visual tasks that were not possible when standing on all fours.

The primate self-identity acquired a tripartite neuronal mechanism that included two older epochs of major forms of life. The primate had deep within its behavior, the older behaviors of first reptiles, and then, the old mammals. With the advent of a more complex vision, primates expanded the self-identity of their predecessors. While primates expanded their sense of self with larger territories (Primate fossiliferous deposits are to be found all over Europe and North America.), it was just an old mammalian mandate. While they maintained hierarchies and fought over mates, they were just acting out their reptilian instincts. With their evolved vision and more intricate motor behaviors associated with that vision, they acquired a new sense of self that became the primitive model for modern humans.

Primate brains provided behavior that diluted what old mammals had diluted from the reptiles. The taste of the solution was still there, but the concentration of the solute was less than it had ever been before. The new self-identity was brought about by the inhibition of older brain organization by newer. It was the visual system of neurons that came to inhibit the neurons of taste and smell not with total paralysis, but only with modification. Primates began the first culture in which animals lived in an extended relative harmony of nuclear families.

Out of the evolving monkey mentality, came the *troupe-state*, a regular community of animal souls that had a special individuality. Yet, they were just a new bud of a tree that sprang from a simple seedling. In contrast to past reptiles that singly fought their own kind as well as predators, and in contrast to past mammals that fought in those same conflicts in twos and threes, primates evolved to fight with small armies. While they retained a monarchy, it was diluted not only to create a warrior class, but also to handle the greater number of females. Subordinates were eventually given rights to ladies by default. The concubines were many and too exhausting for one king to control in a large society. Too many females came into heat at the same time. As the chief primate slept from exhaustion, his rivals did their work with females in readiness. Thus, the beginning of man's future society created its own evils of promiscuity and prostitution. Gangs, brotherhoods of young rivals, arose from the greater numbers as the result of successful survival. Individual families coexisted within the system, but there was a Medici monkey family with one male and his concubines in control of all the other families in a micro society.

To manage this new way of life, primates utilized their new vision to communicate the departure from the reptile's behavior of death to all comers from one sadistic chief. While old mammals had also evolved with sensory mechanisms to avoid such behavior with warning cries of fear and anger, body feints of attack and retreat, the primates evolved more refined visual messages to avoid pain. Enemies and rivals were controlled beyond body injury by using visual mimetic expressions. They began to communicate and express their emotional states of mind primarily with a silent visual language that was passed on to early hominids who also used it as their primary means of expression.

Chapter 5

THE MODEL H

HOW HOMINIDS EVOLVED A GREATER SENSE OF SELF WITH A
GREATER VISUAL MEMORY.

Martin, the Child Paleoanthrope

Looking back on Martin Kaminski's infancy, his troubles seemed
to start there. Martin Kaminski, the firstborn male child to the David
Kaminski family, was unusually busy; he did not border on hyperactivity,
he invaded it and consumed it. His bottle feedings required a trip to the
kitchen sometimes eight or ten times during a night. His parents would
take turns doing this arduous task. They were unable to get relief during
the day because his naps were just momentary fits of inactivity. Martin's
father, David Kaminski, was not too unhappy to escape to the labors of
being a medical student.

Later, Martin's crawling about the floor required constant supervision
to prevent a child induced earthquake of tabletop items falling from
the effects of gravity and agitation from a quadruped below. Once the
transition from four-legged animal ambulation to the human bipedal
form took place even the tables and chairs were in jeopardy. Now they
were threatened by hurricane force impacts from a child's uncontrolled
avalanche-style gait. Martin Kaminski soon was able to be identified in
redeemable family ways as smart and beautiful. He understood diaper
training way ahead of his kind. When he was only two, he could tell
which key was for the front door and which was for the family car. Things
reverted to his perplexing nature when Martin Kaminski was about three

years of age. He developed a bizarre behavior often associated with a febrile illness. He had night terrors. In this children's malady, that some veterans home from Vietnam combat also experienced, a temporary split in Martin's mind occurred. The child's body would respond to positions and actions that appeared as if nothing were wrong. Martin, in an attack of a night terror, would be placed in the tub and soaked to get his temperature down. As he sat there holding a yellow rubber duck, with both his frightened parents beside him to wipe him down, his mind was not there. He was visually fighting, screaming and crying against some terrible force that seemed demonic to those watching. Martin's mind was unable to be awakened but his body was awake. He had split in two parts, one part was a body that worked and the other was a mind that was asleep dealing with devil forces. Within a few minutes, he could again see the real world, glad to be back among those that were in it.

The entire Hominid family has been identified in one way or another for a period that spans over one million years. This immense period of time chronicles the changes in evolution from simian to human that resulted in what we recognize as an animal form, somewhat like monkey, and somewhat like human. While the evolution is a blurred transition in this consideration, what made the hominid "human" occurred in the Middle Paleolithic period 250,000 years ago because of a specific neuronal development. The identifying marker of this evolution of self-identity arbitrarily is assigned to Homo sapiens neanderthalensis, the Neanderthal man. It is appreciated that the slow, imperceptible development of change into a human can best be recognized in him.

The simians, as have been described, evolved from prior epical changes in animal sense of self. Out of single cell membrane definition of self evolved a sense of self that was defined by the surfaces of an animal's body. Then it evolved to a self beyond the body perimeters to a reptilian extension of a body self, a body in a territory within which were hierarchical rivals, mates, prey, dens and upon its borders, predators. This reptilian core of self evolved further in old mammals to extend the limited self-identity of territory to more extensive, migratory territory. Within this larger domain, there evolved a greater inhibition of an aggressive self for mates, offspring, against rivals, pursuing prey and single defense against predators. The simian self developed a further sense of a social community with inhibition of an aggressive self-identity for rivals, mates, pursuing prey, gathering other food and the solo defense against predators.

These great systems of identity were joined together. One did not replace another. The three epochs of self-identity became intertwined. The older forms of identity changed, but kept modified characteristics of the old through that evolution. So it came to pass, a quarter of a million years ago that the hominid self-identity from which humans evolved, came into being. The simian self-identity was genetically bound in hominid brains. Monkey behavior in them, required almost no learning. It was almost automatic. In fact, all the older parts of hominid self-identity combined with those of the reptile and the old mammal were automatic. It was only the last simian component that required learning. (We can now see the self-identity of the family, Hominidae at its beginning.) It had the simian's triune brain with its automatic sense of self-identity, parts of which were ruthlessly reptilian, partly subdued mammalian and socially simian.

After a lengthy time measured in cultural stages of hundreds of thousands of years, something monumental evolved in the hominid's self-identity. It began the evolution of Homo sapiens. The Neanderthal man's brain, specifically the simian visual sensory nerve cells of the visual system of his brain, evolved a new kind of visual memory nerve cell. A group of visual memory neurons developed unlike the earlier evolved visual neurons that stopped stimulating the brain the moment the visual stimulus was "out of sight".[1] This new visual memory neuron could remember the visual stimulus when it was *out of sight*. The new visual memory neurons could stimulate the new breed of hominid after an actual event had transpired. The transpired visual images were of an automatic simian legacy. These were recognizable images of rivals, mates, predators, prey and other food. The new visual memory neurons provided the Neanderthal with a greater survival ability based on the nuclear behavior of reptiles and all of his predecessors. The early hominids, typified by the Neanderthal, extended self-identity with a greater visual memory known as eidetic visual memory in children today.

This new visual memory provided a much greater capability to deal with predators, rivals, to maintain a hierarchy of rivals, to control mating and to defend the territory during the daytime. The new memory had some initial side effects however, that placed Homo sapiens on a narrow-gauge track of precarious and costly mental development. At night, before sleep could be achieved, the new memory of visual images of prey, predators, rivals and mates could not be easily inhibited by the sensory panorama of daylight dependent visual perceptions until the light of a campfire extended daylight. (Even then, as contemporary aboriginals demonstrate, the inhibition is hardly satisfactory.) Neanderthal man's initial use of fire

---

[1]   Alligators are easily subdued as are reptilian derived birds of prey by the use of blinders. Unable to see, these animals with simple visual memory can't remember what they just saw once it is out of sight.

came from volcanic lava or burning trees ignited from lightning. This use of fire during the night for protection occurred at some early period of the Old Stone age. Fire became sacred over ensuing generations of early human development for good prehistoric reasons. These night dependent virtual images of simian realities of daylight stimulated their old mammalian and especially their old reptilian brain parts about predators, prey, rivals and mates. It was especially true if a sound or a smell brought on visual memory. (Contemporary adventurers in Australia's outback have often been entertained by this kind of aboriginal nocturnal cinema.) These images were not dreams, as we now know them; they did not take place after sleep had commenced. They were akin to visual hallucinations that occur in night terrors, certain types of schizophrenia and delirium tremens. These images could evoke all the deep emotions of reptiles, old mammals and simians, especially pain, fear and anger. They could also pacify with gratifying images of mating and food. Nobody needed mescaline, angel's dust or opium. Those things were already in their heads. At night, predatory problems doubled, one was real; another was virtual.

In Ken Wilber's description of the evolution of human consciousness in *Up From Eden*, he quotes Arieti who stated: ". . . (the Neanderthal) . . . would have great difficulty in distinguishing (memory) images and (drawn) paleosymbols from external reality" (I would add in the former, mostly at night, in the latter, only when a real predator didn't steal the show.)

Over time, in the middle Paleolithic stage of man, some of the Neanderthals developed more than the ability to remember visual images of survival significance after they had occurred. Those more intelligent Neanderthals began to draw stick figures and to make crude clay figures. They started drawing on the walls of caves, sedimentary rock cliffs known as respaldos to Mexican archeologists and eventually on stones and animal bones. These were not the artistic renderings we appreciate at Lascoux and Trois Freres as well as other caves of France and Spain from a later period of the Cromagnon, forty to twenty thousand years ago. These first drawings were the evolved appropriate hand-drawn responses to visual memories within the brain. We still see petroglyphs all over North America drawn by New Stone Age man.

The few that learned to draw those childlike figures became very powerful within their clans. They were able to evoke simple emotions and behaviors with those drawings as others did much later with more elaborate Magdalenian drawings and still later, with masks and idols. These few more gifted Neanderthals likely learned to draw stick figures by mimicking and observing objects in nature that simplistically appeared to them as those visual retained images in their brains. They drew and molded with their simian hands.[2]

The relief of a mountain range could represent a sleeping woman as Mt. Tempanocus did for old Ute Indians in central Utah. (There are also those Grand Tetons in Wyoming.) There was a "Y" of a branch that suggested a portion of anatomy and there was a relief of a rock outcropping that looked like a human's facial profile. A palisade of basalt looked like an erect penis. (A cave called San Javier in upper Baja California reveals hundreds of engraved oval figures anthropologists consider vulva symbols carved by New Stone Age man.) While there is conjecture about the reasons these engravings were made, the new memory neurons and the ability to express those almost visual memories in crude drawings, carvings and figures provided a new and powerful way to manage the Neanderthal society. It gave a new mental tool to those in power and created the first shaman, the priest class. There came a new power advantage for survival under the strongest and most fit reptile-old mammal-monkey, the Neanderthal chief. It would be the beginning of brains and not entirely brawn that would come to maintain the social order. Those Neanderthal brains acquiring this new power had only to draw stick figures or present a clay figure to achieve it. They took the power that belonged to nature to make clan members think they could bring about the menstrual cycle and, with symbols, convinced clan members they had helped the gods to achieve it. They could intimidate rivals, subordinates and antagonists beyond tissue injury from direct combat, beyond combat that came close to tissue injury and beyond threats of tissue injury from body actions, to a new intimidation that did not require their physical involvement or presence. It is supposed that early hominids including Neanderthal, used crude hand and arm signs to intimidate and control clan members and antagonists of other clans as well. Hand and finger gestures very likely came about in human interaction before the use of drawn crude stick figures and clay models. But gestures required the presence of the dominant individuals to wield their authority. It is worth considering hand gestures as the beginning of visual language that evolved to stick drawing, cave carvings and eventually into pictorial writing later in the history of civilizations. Retained visual memory associated with hand signs and drawn symbols and clay models was a more evolved sensory-motor brain

---

[2] Early stick figure drawings and later Cuneiform writing was accomplished not as we write today with the thumb and index finger holding a pen, but in early times, the writing stick was held with all four fingers and excluded the thumb.

activity that could serve the survival of Homo sapiens without the prior huge expenditure of life and energy needed to do the same thing.

Initially, the sensory images in the brains of Neanderthal clan members resulted in nocturnal hallucinatory-like impressions. Later, a motor response to the sensory images brought about a drawn primitive replica on rock or in sand. The majority within a clan were activated or held in check by these symbols drawn by a few more sophisticated Neanderthals. Subsequently, one clan with the skill to draw would dominate other clans with only the sensory component of visual memory evolved in their heads. Those with the incomplete sensory-motor visual equipment more easily became the obligatory servants of those with the new brainpower. Slavery and subjugation of tribes and clans began in this ancient process of dependence upon symbolic intimidation as well as physical dominance.

As the visual image memory neurons continued to change the behavior of Paleolithic man, the great cave paintings of Cro-Magnon men emerged thousands of years later. The subject matter was the same, prey, predators, mates and rivals. Now the power-complex of priest-hunter created the earliest organized religion with elaborate drawings. White states: "To manipulate (draw) the symbol (of a bison) by drawing it, by placing a drawn spear in it they (the Cro-Magnon hunter-priests) could affect the object drawn (the bison)." Taylor's work defines ancient man: "in a low stage of mental development, that between the drawn object and the real object there is a real connection." The object in the real world was barely different from the drawn object because it evoked the same simple new visual memory. (Levy-Bruhl's "participation mystique" becomes understandable when we appreciate visual symbolic influences of simple minds.) The Neanderthal leaders of clan hierarchies with their physical dominance and ability to create symbols could control the rest of the clan to respond to their own body postures, facial expressions, arm and hand signs and now with the drawing of signs and stick figures. (This power still exists today in primitive cultures in the form of amulets and fetishes.) Man's self-identity at the time of the Neanderthal was controlled in groups by leaders with special visual drawing skills. The newly evolved brain with the visual motor neurons that could draw, were possessed by a special few. They had the ability to stimulate sensory visual brains that did not have that motor ability. Those early clan members had bodies that were physically separate, but their brains were not separate from their leaders. The newly evolved visual memory was separate, but the ability to manipulate it symbolically with their own drawn figures was only in the brains of a few more advanced members that used their new brain tool to continue the mandates of the triune simian brain even when they were not present to do so by physical means.

The Neanderthal self-identity, that was to become our own, was not males and females in a hierarchy with any sense of equality or individuality, with "minds of their own". The self-identity of those early mind deficient humans was a plural sense of self. There was the parent leader, the male warrior chief or two, what contemporary tribes would consider the elders, and those other maturing rival males and females and offspring.

As a child, you really are your parents. The parents' anger, happiness, pain and fear determine your very own emotions. You wait and watch the parent in order to mimic or respond to his or her behavior. Think about the child playing with its own excrement and seeing the parent reaction. Think about a child watching a parent crying bitterly over a lost relative. The child responds to the stimulus of anger in the parent with its own response of fear. The child responds with its own crying to the visible stimulus of the parent's crying. The Neanderthal clan member's plural mind exists within the relationship of modern parent-child.

All subordinates in the Neanderthal clan hierarchy were not mental individuals, but were mixed up in the head of the chief male. His emotional states of anger, fear, contentment, lust and hunger were mimicked by everyone else. Fight or flight, hunt or be hunted and other responses to simian biological necessity were determined by the modified reptilian monarch, the Neanderthal chief. This behavior of plural self or "clan ego" as Sorenson describes it, occurred because only the chief had a completely developed Neanderthal brain. He was a ten year old in charge of a group of five year olds. Complete development for the Neanderthal meant that a stimulus first in the environment or a retained visual memory of an event in the environment could activate a hand motor response from the chief's brain. It was a complete sensory motor circuit of only his brain. The subordinates were in a slowly developing, in a sense, retarded state of having a complete sensory-motor circuit in their brains. The Neanderthal clan chieftains, the early masters of the clans liked it that way; it kept them in control of the hierarchy. The incomplete state of brain evolution was simply that the stimulus for a body action or a primitive emotional state was in one brain, the chief's. The responses were in the subordinates. (Neanderthal clan member see chief do, Neanderthal clan member do. This behavior is called psycho-motor mimicry by modern psychologists and is highly descriptive of children with developing brains that can only be stimulated by their parents' brains.)

Chapter 6

A Female Voice in the Ancient Wilderness

How the evolution of auditory language began female rights.

Roberta Orensten who would become Mrs. David Kaminski, was raised in a medical doctor's family. As the second born she was the designated beauty of Almar and Mildred Orensten's two daughters. The firstborn was a disappointment. She was intended to be a boy. Roberta went through her early childhood as her own brand of Shirley Temple. Adults and children alike were drawn to her charm and good looks. She was given ample lessons in social etiquettes that she learned to embellish with inviting smiles that got her the attention to demonstrate them. Her rigid maternal education also included a morality that created a dutiful young woman who learned that the body was a thing to adorn not indulge. Miss Orensten was a social force with her attributes long before she entered college to become a beauty queen. There, she was not attracted to macho males even though she dated many of them. Male sexual aggressiveness and egotistical story telling were at odds with the ABC's she lived by. She remained happy within the spiritual love of her chieftain father until the message of her sorority sisters let it be known that one of the main reasons a girl came to college in those days of the 1950's was to get a husband who could provide after graduation.

By chance, Miss Orensten came upon David Kaminski through the formal dating process called an exchange. It was a way for fraternity boys to get to know sorority girls. Kaminski was shy, but subtly humorous. In addition to these traits, Kaminski was attractive to Miss Orensten because he could barely talk about himself. His verbal intercourse seldom started with the pronoun "I". Not understanding her attraction, she took a chance on a long shot who couldn't find the nerve to kiss her after more dates than even she thought appropriate. Kaminski would eventually let it be known he was in pre-medical training in the hope of becoming a doctor. It wasn't a real issue with Miss Orensten. What drove her was a deeper motivation that had something to do with a type of male she felt she could take charge of. Thoughts of achieving a marital union turned into a reality for many reasons, one of which was the reticence of both parties to become sexually viable before marriage. David and Roberta were married a year before he had finished his premedical education and a year after Miss Orensten was hard at work in a department store. Kaminski was a year behind in school, and a year younger than his new wife.

The couple consummated their marital rights with gusto and within just a few years, they had produced three children. The father was still a student but in medical school. The mother was still a young woman hoping her husband would take care of her. Neither had any awareness that the scope of marriage included parenting which would become so emotionally demanding. To avoid the task, David Kaminski could claim greater responsibilities trying to succeed at being a medical student, but his wife could not avoid the brunt of raising three children under five years of age. Taking care of children rather than being cared for was a task only reflex memory of her own mother's behavior could provide.

"You damned brats, what are you kids doing now?" Mrs. Kaminski came upon three children drawing poly-chromed crayon lines over a bedroom wall. A Vulcan's tirade ensued from Mrs. Kaminski. With teeth gritted, she shook each child in turn. A deeply furrowed brow and raised eyelids accompanied the thunderclap of anger. "Sit, sit there, don't move or I'll beat you, do you hear me? Wait until your father comes home and I tell him about this. Don't move until I tell you to, you hear me?" The children remained frozen, it was the way their mother had spoken to them as much as the words she spoke. They could hardly understand words.

Contemporary Stone Age cultures demonstrate to us that most likely very early in Homo history, visual sign language developed a good deal before auditory symbolic language. Sounds create the communication of speaking and listening with symbols, the art of humans talking to one and other. Contemporary primitive savages (we are told from several sources) can barely talk at night, because they are dependent upon facial visual effects to understand their verbal communication. In counting, primitives can only appreciate numbers up to twenty, a process derived from the visualization of toes and fingers. (Today men are considered less communicative than women. They are admired for being strong silent types or disapproved for the same reason.) The sexual differences in verbal communication likely has an ancient etiology.

When primitive clans and tribes divided up the functions of survival, the extended gestation and development of children encouraged a natural division of labor into male-hunters and female-gatherers and child-tenders. Once hunting and gathering stopped being a group activity, mature males did the hunting and females raised the young and performed other domestic functions of gathering. Because of these different tasks, another division arose in the mode of communication. It was prudent for the male-hunters to communicate to each other in visual language and more efficient for female-gatherers to communicate with each other in sound language. Males acquired the art of symbolic visual language and females were not given much of an opportunity to do so. Again, there was a matter of clan dominance the chief male wished to retain. Silence, but the need to communicate in hunting parties, was absolutely necessary for success. Males, pursuing prey, encircling prey, required a visually efficient language of hand, finger and arm symbols. Meanwhile, what was going on back in the den had no such need. It was far more efficient to use sound language to communicate the performance of domestic tasks. Females developed the art of modern sound language, not men. Males, back from the hunt, began to find women talking not with their hands but with their tongues.

Jaynes' work on the origin of auditory language consciousness does not take into consideration that an entire visual symbolic language was in place when auditory symbolic language began to develop. Wilber reviews scholarly evidence of Arieti and Sullivan who describe the first forms of human communication as being both auditory and visual. A "mixture" of the two existed early on for reasons previously identified. The exact time of origin of this mixed communicating can easily be proposed as coming on while man was still a hunter, but fixed in what was the beginning of a Home Land, a fixed territory that would produce not just the meat of prey, but the plenty of vegetable matter women could gather. This occurred at a time somewhere between the Middle Pleistocene and the Upper Pleistocene geological periods. While we appreciate that hand and finger sign language developed a hieroglyphic form of writing and later a cuneiform equivalent and that auditory language evolved a written alphabet from hieroglyphs of sounds, both forms of communication extended the control of human hierarchical groups by the dominant few.

Initially however, the domestic development of auditory symbolic communication created great changes in the reptilian dominance of hierarchies by males. Females acquired their own territory within the territory of the dominant males. The hearth, the keeping of the flame and the control of the den slowly came to be dominated by the females. The "clan ego" of Sorenson, the plural sense of self-identity of early clans was developing a division of that plural wholeness into a sense of female-self within a hierarchical male dominated clan-self. Aural language development initially provided the female of the human species a powerful tool to inhibit the power of males until males better learned auditory symbolic language to dominate further all of those within the clan hierarchy. (The long houses of Borneo's modern day aboriginals are still off limits to females. The males want the boys back to give them a male character that originally included the language of males. Clubs for males in their many modern forms give evidence to the uneasy coexistence of men and women since females took charge of the dens of the territory.)

In their dens, the females reared the male offspring for good physiologic body development. There were also psychological effects of that rearing. Until puberty, the male offspring were as much female as they were male in physical and mental character. They initially modeled after the head mother. The weaning of males at puberty was to inflict a male character on once prepubescent males who identified with females. Prior to this process, however, the females had complete control of the male offspring throughout their early development and these males would be forever bound to the identity of females in some form or other in later life.

While adult males were in their separate environment, females began their control of younger males. Auditory language that developed from newly evolved auditory sensory neurons gave them the same power as male visual language initially achieved. Sound symbols of body commands and imperatives could check undesirable body actions of children. The free flowing visual-motor behavior of monkey-like children could be prevented. Children learned to recognize a command word spoken with the authority of body, facial, arm and hand gestures and with the loudness of anger from the dominant mothers of their clans. These dominant females could speak as well as recognize certain sound symbols that stood for the initiation or inhibition of body acts. The more intelligent females controlled other females and children with the ability both to recognize and to speak symbols while those not so intelligent could only recognize those symbols. Again, it was a situation in which those less intelligent females and children first could only understand auditory symbols, only the few more intelligent females could both speak and understand auditory symbols. Males, with their visual symbolic control over their hierarchies, were not far behind in appreciating that auditory language was a power they could not allow to go uncontrolled. Males were developing, then, with the language of their mother's tongue. Those males that learned to speak the new auditory language were to wrest control of the hierarchy and the territory from those males that could communicate only with visual symbols. That change would dramatically reveal itself in the Neolithic period when farming and group laboring on things not the hunting of animals demanded a greater efficiency in communication that aural symbolic language would easily provide.

Chapter 7

TO BE OR NOT TO BE

HOW THE EVOLUTION OF AURAL LANGUAGE RESULTED IN THE
HUMAN DUALISTIC SENSE OF SELF.

"Come and get this damned dog, I can't take it any longer." Dr. Kaminski, completely exasperated, was calling his wife long distance from their cabin in the San Juan Islands of the State of Washington. "I have too much I want to do to spend all day changing this dog's diapers." The new poodle, Black Jack, was just a puppy; he was entering the human world that demanded urination in some places but not in others. It turned out to be a difficult assignment for the puppy to learn and his master to teach.

The poodle could not develop into the full-blown expression of the dog genus. He could not fight to become the Alpha male, mount a female in heat or become a member of a pack chasing down an old, dying bison. Black Jack was to be stunted in his natural development. He was to become man's best friend and his obedient servant. While he was becoming domesticated, people would spot him from across a street and come with out-stretched hands just for a feel of his glossy hair-like coat. Babies would find a new reason to smile with their first sight of him. His meager training did not prevent him from rising easily to deserve the claims that he was one of the most intelligent of the species. He quickly learned to understand Dr. Kaminski's verbal commands, sit, stay, fetch, go find Momma (Mrs. Kaminski), go get baby (his furry doll,) and many other words, but Black Jack never learned to speak the human language. In his little brain, he could understand a number of words his master spoke. When he heard them, he knew just what body action he was to perform. When it came time to come in from out of doors, he could only bark. But it wasn't long before Dr. Kaminski recognized a specific bark that said, "I want to come in now."

Black Jack and the hominids that just preceded Homo sapiens thousand of years ago had something in common. Black Jack and all domesticated dogs still are, and hominids were, language deficient. Before language became accessible to all humans we must appreciate just a few gifted individuals could both speak and understand aural language. In that distant past, most humans did not have a developed left cerebral language cortex in their brains. In fact, the world over, there were many tribes of early humans that existed side by side with other tribes of humans that first could not even understand aural language. The gradual and bumpy evolution of language provided for a distribution of humans that had no auditory language and those that could both understand and speak verbal language. This distribution of using auditory symbols in communication does not include the understanding of sounds with an emotional character. All hominids prior to the acquisition of symbolic language could appreciate emotional sounds.

The relationship between Black Jack and his master held true for the dominant speaking clan male or female and their clan members. (While dog and master are certainly separate physical bodies, part of the dog's brain can only be activated by the vocal motor action of his master's brain.) In the same manner, most hominids acquiring language had only a sensory or receiving part of their brain for aural language. They did not have a motor or sending part of their brain for that language. The complete development of a brain that could send and receive took an immense length of time to be acquired by all. During that lengthy period, incomplete language utilization was common for many people.

Language created a new self-identity for Homo sapiens and a new power for those that controlled groups of early humans. As symbolic language evolved in the human, each new development of language was used to control those in hierarchical clans and tribes. There was first the visual-language dominant male and those that were bound to him and to his territory. Then there was a division of survival of labor in which gender determined that labor. In time, men hunted and women kept the den, suckled the young and created a second sub-hierarchy of females who developed their own language. This breakdown of the male dominated clan ego accompanied by a second language did not provide for a greater self-identity for each individual. The extent of brain individuality that did develop was a division of the larger heterosexual survival group into sexual identification, not just by body differences, but also through language differences. It is important to keep in mind that prior evolution of cells into body-organisms with a nervous system that identified the extent of the body-organism gave each and every mature member of a prehistoric clan a body sense of individuality. When early Homo sapiens of the middle Paleolithic culture stuck his finger in the fire, he knew exactly where his body began and ended. Early man had a sense of body-self, but his sense of mind-self was undifferentiated from a dominant clan leader. Early members of clans were neurologically bound to the leader's control of their bodies. Clan members had no will to use their bodies beyond the direction of their dominant leaders.

What the headman or woman did, the clan members would do. When the head-person felt anger or fear, the clan members would also feel those very same emotions. Then, with the evolution of language, clan members could "read" their chiefs with symbols in addition to the emotional sound of their voices. Clan members had separate bodies that they well appreciated were separate, but they had no such separate minds. An infamous German patriarch in more recent times intuitively knew the importance of this ancient history when he made the German army swear allegiance to him, not to the Fatherland. Hitler's regressive command to his soldiers acknowledged the inseparability of the reptile kingdom and early man's obligatory behavior that evolved from it. We can understand that those in control of early forms of auditory language shunned letting their hierarchical members learn the skills of speaking verbal language. It became part of their armamentarium of power.

In addition to observations of domesticated animals, humans learning a second auditory language today provide insight into how language evolved in our brains. There is a fundamental process of language that reflects the nature of the entire central nervous system. You first must hear a language spoken before you can learn to speak it. There is first a sensory comprehension that results in a motor action, there is listening and then there is speaking. (Early language development was a language likely of imperatives, of commands for whole body action. "Stop", "run", "come", "sit", "stay" were words tied to whole body motor acts. The individual speaking the command was in control of the recipient who had just imprinted the sensory word symbol in his auditory sensory cortex. Soon after, the word became wired in the brain to a motor act. It was an obligatory neurological connection only life threatening events could begin to check.) Marine drill instructors have intimidated recruits to behave like prehistoric men. They are outside of the recruits' brains, stimulating them with words on which to act. The recruits are allowing the brains of drill instructors to take control of their body actions. "Esprit de corps" is a military term that refers to a training process to break down an individual's will by taking away his individual self-identity and to mold it back into an ancient sense of group self-identity. It begins with the drill sergeant who is given absolute authority.

Less intelligent, less evolved prehistoric men for many generations could only understand language sounds, not everyone could speak. Those that could do both controlled those that had not developed both capabilities. They kept the control from childhood to adulthood, from generation to generation. They inhibited language development in clan members in order to control them. ("Tell grandmother your name. Go get your new doll. Sing a song. Put your shoes on." These words we speak to children learning to speak, are examples of someone in command telling someone else what to do with his body. We allow our children to continue on with language and speak it back to us as a matter of course, but that was not the case in prehistoric times.) The prehistoric Homo developing language had not learned to say, "No, I don't want to." He was still partly in the brain of his master for life not just during his childhood. His early language was just doing what his body was told to do by his master.

What early man was told to do with his body by those that knew how to speak words was dependent upon the visual and auditory physical presence of the hierarchical master. The brain arrangement of being part in their own brains and part in their master's necessitated that member of clans were in a very close mental and physical union, within ear shot, within sight of the master. They continued to have a plural self-identity bound to one and another doing tasks and behaving in unison.

This theory holds that object names came soon after commands in language of early man. "Catch deer. Kill deer." The advancement of language vocabulary continued to maintain control of clan members' bodies to perform specific tasks on specific things with names. Jaynes concludes that the names of individual humans came late in language evolution. What came first, before individual names, likely was the personal pronoun "you". Everybody was called you. You run. You sit. You spear. You hunt. Everybody looked up to see if the "you" referred to a few individuals rather than the whole group. It would only be determined by the pointing of the visible finger of the chief. In English, we continue to use the word "you" for one person or twenty persons. "You" was the further breakdown of clan plural identity. The new word signaled the evolution of greater individuality into groups to perform more specific tasks within the clan. Separate tasks created more subordinate hierarchies within the sexual division of the hierarchies. The clan chiefs still held control of each individual within his territory as long as each individual was not out of sight or not out of hearing his voice.

When tasks took sub-groups of the clan out of sight, out of voice control, there was hell to pay; the tasks were often not performed until a new sensory auditory neuron also evolved as it had for vision. This new auditory sensory neuron was able to retain in memory the voice symbols even when those symbols were not actually being spoken, even when those that spoke them were not visible. Again Jaynes points out that a retained memory of a voice command would continue to direct humans when away from the physical presence of the clan chiefs. Those humans that were developing this new voice memory, as Jaynes describes, were hearing in their heads auditory voice sounds similar to hallucinations, big, real human voices. The masters were in their heads even when those masters were not really around. The clansmen heard voices that directed them to perform certain tasks not unlike certain psychotics today are driven by internal voices not thought to be their own.

Great power from auditory language was given to primitive humans to extend their core reptilian behavior of dominance over others. The power elite held this new brainpower closely at hand. It was not spread to the clan with any gusto. ("Don't speak until you're spoken to. Silence is golden. A child should be seen and not heard. The fight for the freedom of speech . . ." can all be understood because those originally empowered with speech would not share it with the rest of the clan.) Later in ancient history, those in power of clans that became larger aggregations of humans continued to manipulate the derivatives of speech, reading and writing. These new communication tools were disseminated very slowly to the common man. Until the sixteenth century, only a small number of individuals could both read and write. Chartier tells of the general hostility to writing by the lower classes because writing was the medium in which the decisions of authority were couched. The written word was the instrument of lawyers and royal writs from which complaints submitted to the king and decisions based on them were handed down to local sheriffs. Writing was used to record the obligations of the poor. It was a powerful tool denied the common man.

Tasks performed out of sight and out of the sound of a human voice needed to be verified by the controllers of clans. This new specialized task behavior created the human need for a language of time. When in sight or sound of other humans, those in charge could easily verify the tasks were being done. Questions, as interrogative words or sentences in language, were not necessary when clans worked as groups doing the same tasks. Once tasks were out of sight and out of the sound of a human voice, a word for what had been done or was going to be done became necessary. Questions came into man's vocabulary simply by changing the way the word sounded. "Going" and "going?" are different just by the way they are spoken. Questions made evident by voice inflection opened the way to language that implied time in the form of a future or past tense vocabulary. We don't ask: "Are you at work now?" when the haggard task performer comes back into the camp after a long day of labor. Language had to transcend actual visual and auditory reality of the present to verify events of the past or the future. "Did you work yesterday or are you going to work tomorrow?" are indications of a greater understanding of time than the cycle of the full moon. Time concepts in language of future and past created a second symbolic reality for the human.

Wilber supports the studies of Piaget and Hall in this regard that language begot the idea of time, but not just time for time's sake, but for people being accounted for in the past or future. When the tribal leaders acquired primitive auditory or visual language, they did not appreciate its symbolic nature. In the beginning of language, it was a matter of conditioning object events of reality in terms of other senses to individual sounds. Then the realness of symbols acted as strongly on human actions as did the objects the symbols stood for. The responses appeared to be the same as the Pavlovian experiments tell us.

With the new vocabulary that included past and future, tribal leader-priests also began story telling to their followers. They created a symbolic world we now know as mythology. "Then the Raven took Little Beaver up into the sky and that is how we came to honor our ancestors and mind the rules of our forefathers." There was no way to disprove these stories; there was no need to do so because symbolic reality and objective reality were indistinguishable. Chiefs and priests could say whatever they wanted about the future and the past. What was said about past or future events was a new means of controlling those not in the priesthood. The priests eventually could prove time by demonstrating the accurate appearance of celestial bodies that confirmed their power of past and future. Physical seeing, touching, smelling, tasting, and hearing of reality were verifiable in every day life, but the past and the future were very different. To predict a physical thing that could be verified gave magical power. In the beginning of this development of language, the word symbols spoken about past and future events could go without any other form of verification. The primal chiefs took advantage, once again, of a brain evolution that created through language vocabulary, the concepts of past and future. The symbolic idea of past and future through language vocabulary evolution created not only a new mental world that could not be verified by the senses, but also a new way of controlling and binding followers to their leaders.

While manipulating and controlling their members with mythical past or future reality that could not be verified except by the priests, the primal chiefs would not allow such a reality to exist in their tribal members. Tribal leaders forbade talking among clan members unless the talking served the clan's purpose. Early language developed in clan members in spite of leaders' attempts to prevent it from happening. Leaders, nonetheless, tried to block common use of all new language developments such as the vernacular of future and past words of time. Future and past language usage would allow the members of clans too much freedom. Talking about what had happened or what was going to happen was for the chiefs and priests. If used by the tribe members, it would allow them to exist not only in the present, but also in the unverifiable past and future. They would be out of control just by using certain word symbols.

A tribal member once out of sight and coming out of the obligatory verbal and obviously visual control of his master could do what his body wanted to do. The body, controlled by its monkey-hominid brain, wanted to do exactly the opposite of what the master wanted it to do. It wanted to follow its simian instincts: sleep, eat, fornicate, kill and take for its body-self. As the tribal member developed his own motor language skills of talking, he began talking back to authority out loud, (the only way he could), when the boss could not hear him. He began to obstruct voice commands stuck in his head. He could then commit crimes against the tribe or act independently. When individuals acted against the clan, the clan leaders had to prove those crimes had taken place. They had to maintain control for the clan's sake which was indistinguishably their own.

Early members of clan and tribal hierarchies eventually acquired the new future-past language skills of their manipulating masters in spite of their objections. What the subordinate clan member said he had done was true until it was proven otherwise. Primitive man did not actually lie because in the beginning of the use of future-past language all virtual language subjectivity was as real as object reality. He eventually learned to lie to cover his cheating, stealing and indolence when confronted with punishment. The tribe leaders could not trust tribal members that learned the new future and past forms of language. What the tribal member said and what he did were often two different realities. Thousands of years later even American primitives were confounded by white men talking with forked tongues. The chiefs of prehistoric tribes established punishment for those that had those two tongues. The mind that speaks must represent the body that acts. In simple tribal communities, punishment was not necessarily handed out to one person, often the entire tribe was punished for one individual's crime. In nineteenth century Europe, the process continued. It was commonplace for family members of incarcerated German criminals to go to a separate prison as well.

Chapter 8

THE EVOLUTION OF THINKING

HOW THE AUDITORY LANGUAGE BRAIN (THE MIND) EVOLVED TO
CREATE MORE POWER FOR CLAN LEADERS AND EVENTUALLY A
PLACE FOR CLAN MEMBERS TO HIDE.

In a childhood without siblings, David Kaminski longed for visits from his favorite cousin, Delbert Kaminski. Delbert lived in Salt Lake City with his two brothers and his divorced mother. Still trying to prop up an only child, David's parents invited Delbert into their home in Spokane, Washington each summer. Delbert was intended to be a counter social force to shyness and introversion in the role of foster brother. Delbert's father, Fillmore Kaminski, was David's paternal uncle who escaped the manacles of the LDS church and its oppression, not by flight or submission to Mormon doctrines, but by the numbing effects of alcohol. Fillmore was a housepainter when he wasn't tippling or falling from his equipment.

Delbert lived with his mother in a substantial poverty. His visits to Spokane resulted in new clothes and new demands from his father's patriarchal older brother. Delbert's visits provided both reward and punishment especially for Mrs. Kaminski who was determined to "fix" David's shyness which had started well before he was eight years old. It abruptly came to Mrs. Kaminski's attention, however, that Delbert had problems of his own; he was a bed wetter. Uriniferous wet sheets were assaulted with frequent nocturnal visits to the bathroom. Sleep deprived, Delbert still began to provide a social atmosphere that awakened David out of the daydreaming that was his substitution for social intercourse.

Nonetheless, Delbert's infrequent visits were only mildly successful in creating the art of social interaction. David fought shyness most of his life. During piano recitals, dissonance mistakenly produced within the most melodic of John Thompson's piano studies revealed his early stage fright. Spelling tests in a room of second grade competitors often caused him to place an "e" before an "i". Any future activity that required a self-confidence to perform brought on the terror of the condemned about to die. Ringing wet with ochlophobia he was a timid thespian and orator. Later on in life, his muted character vanished into thin air when he tried a couple swigs of beer. He then became known, quite surprisingly, as a "motor mouth". David's retarded ability to speak out with words was accompanied by a physical reticence to move his body with any ease or fluidity. His early performances on various athletic fields reminded coaches of a newborn herd animal trying to stand upright. But David had some resources; there was the drumming in his head from his father that kept the beat of "Don't be a quitter, no matter what!". He also had his fantasies that envisioned his gawky body, agilely twisting and turning, cloaked in a basketball uniform numbered "7". In his anticipated role of an athletic Peter Pan, he wished for the adoration of those eating popcorn on the pine rows of seats in the city armory. Through determination and wish fulfillment, David eventually unraveled the coordination problems of most of his muscles except for those that moved his tongue in speech. Much later, as a physician, he preferred to be seen and not heard by staying out of the front row action of the vocally intelligent. When it was necessary to speak in public, he spent long hours memorizing word for word a speech that gave exposition to his ideas, but the memorization could be derailed with the slightest cough in the audience. David looked upon public speaking before three or a hundred individuals as the same; it was a punishment for a crime he couldn't remember, but one he felt he might have committed. It took years before he learned to overcome his early fears, but eventually he began to think on his feet.

Auditory thinking developed from the newly evolved speech sensory and motor neurons in the left cerebral cortex of the Genus Homo. Those neurons, we recall, provided him with the ability to talk and listen to auditory sounds that stood for real objects identified by his other senses. Those neuron clusters in lobes of the brain's left hemisphere evolved to provide first vocal language and then later to create our ability to think in aural symbols. It is important to appreciate that speculation is not unreasonable that the reptilian genetic code of survival would continue to utilize every new development in the brains of humans. The process of thinking and the origins of ideas from thinking are no exception.

Whether originating from the earlier right (visual) hemisphere or the modern left (auditory) hemisphere, the older behavior still persisted.

In this neuron derived theory of the evolution of auditory thinking, it is proposed that in the left cerebral hemisphere of certain more evolved humans, auditory sensory neurons began to recognize certain sounds in nature that occurred with the simultaneous recognition of certain visually identifiable phenomena. Those sounds are what we call today *onomatopoetic* sounds. "Bang, boom, hiss and cuckoo" are examples. When early man heard those sounds they also triggered into action his newly acquired visual memory cortex that could retain visual images long after they stopped stimulating the retina. With his newly evolved visual memory, in his head, he virtually could see the bird that gave out the sound "cuckoo", even when it was out of sight. With his monkey-like ability to mimic sounds and to move his simian acquired mimetic muscles, he was able to make that sound with his own voice. (As we recall, primitive Stone Age people are experts at mimicking birdcalls and animal sounds to lure prey.) Those sounds became retained in the auditory sensory cortex and motor neurons once stimulated by those special memory sensory auditory neurons could alter the larynx, the tongue and the mouth to imitate those sounds. Vocabularies evolved beyond visual signs used in hunting by males. Word vocabularies developed with greater ease by females working closer together and doing tasks that were facilitated by verbal language. Less skilled early humans, as already pointed out, could be controlled by voice symbols from those who could say the new words, because the less skilled could neither say the words back to the speaker, nor could they block the action with the forbidden word "no". Those more skilled humans who could say the new word symbols began to talk, at times not to others, but to themselves when others were not present. Words were "hot stuff", having to do with emotional earthy matters in the beginning. These individuals could make running commentary on actual visual or other sensory impressions as they came upon them. This talking when no one else was around was mostly visually oriented and often rambling, non linear, without grammar as we know it; something today we call flight of words or inane chatter. The talk out-loud was in reference to whatever those individuals saw or whatever visual memories of vital needs popped into their minds. Initially talking was all out loud. Out of one mouth and not necessarily into another's ear but back into the individual's own ear.

Old Stone Age groups of women would eventually acquire the ability to talk out loud to themselves. Working at their special tasks, they must have exhibited a raucous cacophony of human voices, but when others were not present, thinking began to happen out loud. When the dominant female of a prehistoric sub-hierarchy in a clan, began talking to herself without others around, this became the basis of a greater kind of talking we now can consider primitive auditory thinking. When the head female who could both talk and understand words was alone, she spoke commands that were heard in her own auditory sensory cortex. She essentially was stimulating herself. Certain gifted individuals were receiving and understanding the auditory stimulation out of their own mouths. They were listening to themselves talk.

We know people just like that today. They enjoy hearing themselves talk out-loud. They continue to think out-loud as primitives once did learning to think. ("I was saying to myself just the other day, Jolene, why don't you get the kids and spend some time at the zoo?") Jolene is talking to Jolene. The sensory neurons of speech begin to stimulate motor neurons of speech in one head. Neuro-anatomy reveals to us that there are two basic areas for speech in the left cerebral hemisphere for this synaptic interaction to occur. One is sensory and the other is motor.

With more evolution of auditory sensory neurons, it became possible for the sensory neurons to stimulate the motor neurons in less than a talking out-loud mode we appreciate as mouthing or mumbling, under your breath. It was a primitive way of speed talking to yourself. The lips were barely moving, but still moving to form words that were not quite audible. Eventually, in speech evolution, the sensory neurons evolved to stimulate the motor neurons and also inhibit their function on the motor organs of speech altogether. Speech went underground. In reality, a higher order of sensory-motor neurons developed. (You could talk to yourself without making any sounds others could hear. What gives this theory of silent talking that became the process of thinking validity is derived from a similar process that is referred to as silent reading. However, before any reading can be done, there must exist some system of written symbols to be deciphered.)

Initially, writing developed from the glyphs drawn or carved in stone. Drawing signs and symbols were the motor expressions of visual impressions retained in the memory of the right hemisphere. In the beginning, drawing was the only means of communicating these sensations to anyone not present to observe the rudimentary hand signs. Subsequently, thinking in primitive pre-auditory visual Homo was a form of drawing a symbol of a simple object of vision first, and then, a complex idea of vision. For primitive man, who was completely in his right visual hemisphere, drawing was the means of communicating "big ideas". (Even today, charts, graphs, photographs, drawings and computer generated models are intermixed in power-point presentations to illustrate new discoveries, ideas and theories.)

Visual thinking first started in the right hemisphere as reflected in ancient petroglyphs and cave drawings, but then with the advent of a more fluid, more accurate way of talking with auditory symbols, thinking evolved in the left hemisphere as well. As an evolutionary process, auditory thinking evolved first by talking out loud to others, then by talking to oneself (primitive thinking) and finally, by talking (thinking) internally to oneself. Eventually these ideas had to be expressed in a written language.

The development of writing systems varied greatly from civilization to civilization. In ancient Egypt, hieroglyphic writing in which figures or objects were used to represent words or ideas was an adaptation of the prehistoric petroglyphic drawings. Even though the Egyptians had developed an oral language, their writing system retained the visual representations of the past. In Sumer, Babylonia, and Persia, the written language also began as pictographic like the Egyptian system, but altered over time to a cuneiform system of wedge shaped characters which represented words, syllables and letters of an alphabet. This change may have reflected a shift in thinking from the visual right hemisphere to the auditory left hemisphere and the scribes of these early civilizations needed a more efficient way "to spell out" their thoughts. Nowhere is the evolution of the pictograph more evident than in the intricate characters of the oriental writing system, in which one added line or deleted flourish could change one symbol to another or a noun to a verb. We see that in the oriental system the visual hemisphere continued to control the individual and his society and further evolved into a complex ideographic way of thinking and writing. The Rosetta Stone was not only a milestone in our ability to understand the ancient Egyptian glyphic writing but also marked a significant event in evolution in which the right and the left brains met up with their writing descendants from east and west.

Long before the discovery of the Rosetta Stone, however, some men were able to read aloud in one or more languages. During the Middle Ages, one small group after another mastered the technique of silent reading. They were the copyists, working in the monastic scriptoria. The process slowly spread to the lay aristocracy. Before that, reading was all out loud. Reading out loud required groups of listeners. The internalization of reading was a neurological development akin to the internalization of speaking. It required a long history of development. New neurons enabled the simple sensory motor processing of symbolic sounds and symbolic visual images to go from one part of the brain to another without going outside of the brain and back into it. The mouth and the external ear were bypassed.

This bypassing neurological process was the second phase of real thinking. It could take place without others knowing about it. Thoughts were auditory symbols that passed back and forth from just one owner's sensory cortex to his motor cortex without being directed to or heard by any other human ear. It obviously could be a very dangerous thing for tribal leaders if their members started thinking. To be certain, thinking vexed early leaders of city-states and was challenged severely by the early religions including the Christian church. Men died for thinking what they were forbidden to think. But thinking could not be restrained; it allowed man to become his individualistic self no matter to what hierarchy his body and his public words were chained. Yet it was difficult to put individual thinking into action. To say out loud contrary things you thought created peril. You could be burned at the stake.

We can further appreciate the importance of the press that took the power of thinking with written words out of the hands of authority. The scribes of living god-priests and power aligned religions were to be stripped of this power over the commoner. Leaflets and pamphlets of forbidden ideas could be burned, but their authors could survive.

Thinking began as a human characteristic for the very few, yet like writing and reading, it could not help but spread to the masses. In a similar way the newer fruits of thinking, the computers, have spread from the very few of corporate power to the common man. While all humans can't read and write, all humans who have accessed speech think, but the thinking is not uniform from culture to culture, and indeed, within each culture. Its variability is related to how many of each anthropologic group has achieved the most evolved form of thinking. Thinking has its own evolution. Initially, it begins with talking out loud and the repeating out loud what others have said. This is the lowest form of thinking in Bloom's Taxonomy, the simple recall of facts. Once thinking becomes internal or silent, it can be mystical, religious, analytical, rational or scientific. Dictionaries are updated regularly in an attempt to keep up with new words that express current ideas and technologies derived from new ways of thinking and communicating.

Listen to the Socratic silent dialogue of an early thinker. It requires a vocabulary that includes questions of how, where, when, and why. These are words of early analytical thinking. The student and teacher are in one head with a sensory (listening) and motor (talking) cortex in different brain places but in just the left side of the brain. "How can you tell me if this effulgent and lustrous piece of metal is all gold or if it has some other metal within it?" The sensory cortex has stimulated the motor cortex to ask the question, all in one head. The sensory cortex listens to its own question after it was spoken internally by the motor cortex. The sensory cortex recalls all of its auditory memories and directs memory to come forth from all of the brain's other senses. Words, groups of words, scripts of conversations, retained visual experiences, retained visual symbols, smells, tastes and touch memories are accessed and scanned for the answer. Then the sensory cortex tells the motor cortex to tell the answer that now is in the sensory cortex neurons ready to be expressed. The auditory sensory cortex neurons stimulate the auditory motor cortex neurons to talk back to itself. This is a literal example of the process that neurologist Damasio refers to as brain cross talk. The answer to the "gold question" may be as simple as, "I remember having a bath that day in March. The water rose in the tub less after I had lost weight. Things sink into the water differently depending upon their density."

Thinking is not just a process of our auditory symbolic hemisphere going back and forth between sensory and motor neurons in the left side of the brain. It is much more complex because it involves other components of the brain as well. Answers may not always come from just retained verbal recollections of the past. It may come in the darkness of night when only the inspiration of the dreaming visual brain is able to muster the answer for the auditory brain. Dubois tells of these unorthodox origins of thinking we call original ideas. "The idea of the mirror galvanometer occurred to William Thompson (Lord Kelvin), at a moment when he noted a reflection of light from his monocle. The theories of the structure of the atom and of the benzene ring were formulated by Kekule while partially asleep when he could see visions of atoms dancing in his head. Some of the most remarkable discoveries of men, like Gauss, Poincare and Einstein come from a sudden 'illumination'."

The metaphoric use of light is very appropriate because the complex process of thinking involves not just the recollection of retained information on the left hemisphere, but more importantly, information from the right visual hemisphere. Insights and new ideas come from pictures in our right hemisphere and they must be transformed into words by the left. There must be a thorough interaction between both hemispheres in the process of thinking to be "brilliant". While auditory thinking is linear and defining, visual thinking is synergistic to use Carl Jung's terminology. One is reductive while the other is expansive; one is time oriented while the other is timeless. Each on its own is incomplete and for each human being, there must be a balance between right and left thinking to be completely intelligent.

No matter how varied ideas are and from where in the brain they come, they all must be expressed by man's auditory and visual symbolic brain. In the beginning, thinking by a commoner was strictly forbidden. It was too powerful a tool of independence from the hierarchy. Those in

45

charge wanted to hear every word and only the words they put in the heads of their subjects. You were guilty if you even thought certain thoughts; you were not just guilty because you acted upon those thoughts. Torture racks were popular to get those subversive thoughts out in the open so that real punishment could be administered. Thinking was sanguinary stuff. It was much worse than using the simple language of the future and past. There is a price that cultures must pay until humans evolve to be not just what they say they are, but also what they are afraid to say they are. The mind must come to grips with its visual right half. It must unite with it by exposing the hidden visual half in words. It must allow that half of us to develop fully in order to avoid being the next missing link of human survival.

PART II

Introduction

In the early years of his marriage, David Kaminski, in spite of all his ponderous introspection, did not understand why his feelings and behavior were so influenced by what others said. The utterance of a few words could incite a fistfight or the desire to get a divorce. Cutting remarks were as real as the pain he recalled as an adolescent trying to hold his breath for a record of four minutes underwater. When his wife castigated his asocial behavior by saying he was just like his father, the comment was a searing insult but maybe true. When his mother had his fortune read at five years of age, what the gypsy scrutinized in his small right hand, he held onto, never forgetting what appeared to be a prophesy from some pagan oracle. The directive influence of hearing things from others included distant stony commands from his father looking down on his feeble efforts to paint a water color picture of a house. "Change that line. Where is the direction of the light? Do it over again." Taking the tip of the brush out of his seven year old son's mouth, he bent further down, eye to eye, and said: "Don't be a quitter. Do it." And David Kaminski so instructed, thereafter held onto solving tasks until the issues died in the process.

Over the years that followed his childhood, the persistence of those imbedded imperative recollections were defining of his character. In a new adolescent environment, he was easily influenced and got into trouble with bad company. He was living out a selfless dependency upon others because of his father's stern directives that produced inferiority and guilt. With the introduction into the psychiatric aspects of his medical training, he pathetically saw himself in every neurotic patient, not personally, but in an impression of pity for others. However, patients eventually provided him with an objectification of his emotional problems. Finally as a mature physician faced with trying to help others in a medical practice, the process of separating himself from the directives of others slowly came about. He began to see his faulty self and deal with it, like a snake ridding itself of old skin.

It seemed simple in retrospect, because it just came down to the ability to say no. Yet the learning process involved years of painful self-analysis. He looked back and knew it had been a monumental struggle. For many years, Kaminski had been his emotions, a fearful, intimidated, wounded, sulking child. He was initially not conscious that his emotions were only part of his mind, a very old part at that. In those formative years, he could not say, "I felt frightened inside." He was his emotions before developing a mind that appreciated he was more than those emotions which he could control. Kaminski had gone through a process of mind maturation that recapitulated what the human species had passed through in the process of trying to understand itself. He was studying himself and what had changed in that self. He was part of mankind's evolution of trying to understand itself from prehistoric times when it appreciated the primal spirit world. It took a profound attention to what past humans thought of themselves. It involved hindsight and speculation as well as the recorded history of what man thought the self was. For Kaminski, the study of himself was not just egocentric and selfish indulgence, but a need to be in step with the history of man's own soul searching. It was a way of expunging the demons of self-doubt.

The human curiosity of what it is to be human has a long evolution of its own; it's more than a history because the process is hidden in the brain and one that long precedes verbal and written documentation. But the appreciation of the nature of the beast in its natural history, its progression through recorded time, is always participating in a game of catch-up. The study of human self-identity is always one step behind the ever-evolving nature of man's nervous system. (By the time it was figured out that we behave a certain way due to the movements of the celestial bodies in regulated horoscopes, some new thinker, after studying peas growing in his garden, claimed it really was due to a thing called heredity.) The human brain evolves with greater intelligence, but the ability to appreciate changes in our nature is very slow to follow. In that regard, the human that spent his afternoons knapping flint arrowheads is fundamentally related to the gentleman in the gray flannel suit of today. Yet, the two humans are quite different in many ways, especially how they think about themselves. "I had a rush of adrenalin," says the pro football player about to begin a game. Stone Age man did not think that way about being excited.

Likely the early human appreciation of a self had a prehistoric beginning that embraced a primitive mental awareness about the consequences of dying. What was different between a live body and a dead one? The origin of a simplistic awareness of a spirit-body-self beyond other animals, was derived only within the evolving brain of certain bipedal mammals. Their brains alone acquired a neuronal ability to create such a comprehension. Something evolved in the visual brain of those early humans that caused them to appreciate spirits. The comprehension of a world of animism was simplistic, primitive and inaccurate. It was an explanation, in spite of those characteristics, that continues to influence our thinking today. Spirituality determined the character of early man's understanding about a self; it resulted in the near infinite forms of religions many of which persist today. When the evolution of the auditory hemisphere caught up with the visual hemisphere eons ago, a brain development occurred to retain in memory auditory symbols we call words. Those advanced sounds of symbolic memory begot their own progeny that eventually evolved the brain function of thinking. Once the human brain acquired the ability to think, those that did it especially well, splintered away from those that kept to understanding the self in terms of the spirit and its separate body. Those early humans were thought of as a special kind of wise man, separate from the temples of worship; we now recognize them as philosophers with their own schools of thought. They appeared in our recorded history as post Socratic individuals who defied older thinking about the self in terms of spirits, gods and their actions on humans. The brain evolution that resulted in thinking created a new sense of self through a process of theorizing that thrived on evidence. "They began the further study of being outside of the imperative thoughts of spiritualism and the theological creeds that followed." Zenophanes set things on a new course: "Man is not a plethora of gods, the gods of Homer and Hesoid are absurd. There is a single god and a single me."

Philosophical investigations were swept off their feet by a new ability and a new Hellenistic freedom to think outside the scope of religion. With the omnipotence of their new mind-tool, the pursuits of philosophers splurged in every direction to develop the physical sciences that included the study of the human body and the sciences that could cure it of disease.

Yet the look in at the self was circumspect and randomly approached by the parade of new thinkers until Franz Brentano created the science of psychology in 1874. Like a ripe plum it fell from the tree of philosophy to start its own growth. Yet it remained hindered by its spiritual past that kept body and mind separate.

Chapter 1

The Spirit Is Born

How prehistoric man came to believe a spirit was his first self.

David Kaminski timidly peered down at his maternal grandmother's corpse. On tip-toes, he did not dare place his hands on the edge of her open casket to get a better look. Knickers covered but did not disguise knobby knees bouncing off one and another in the rhythm of a flamenco dancer's castanets. A loving mother took his hand and whispered: "She's gone to heaven." just as his aunt Evelyn leaned down into that velvet pink conveyance of passage and kissed grandmother on her wood hard lips.

This scene every human in some way or another must experience. A child must be introduced to the spirit concept of life. Each child, no matter what religious belief it acquires, gets an indoctrination into death. Kaminski's mother explained: "There are two grandmothers, honey." Kaminski could not look at the one in the coffin any longer. The corpse was as ashen as the disgorged mantle of Mt. St. Helen's cataclysm. Her pallor was contested by an Elizabeth Arden body powder but made worse by the contrast of cheeks painted with rouge from the Walgreen Drug Store of Provo, Utah.

The idea was presented to young Kaminski in the granite of ageless wisdom that it was grandmother's body in the coffin, but her spirit, the real grandmother, had departed and was enthroned with Mormon angels in heaven. Married for eternity to Granddad Bourne already there, her spirit would become intertwined with his. Kaminski wondered if his granddad was still wearing his LDS underwear with those funny holes over his nipples. He wondered which star in the heavens his grandfather was now. He later wondered if his granddad's star was as big as the stars up there that were once early Christian martyrs. Still later, he had to remind himself that Mormons were Christians, too.

In August 1908, three abbes, A. and J. Bouys-Sonie and L. Bardon were engaged in a sacrilegious activity. They were investigating traces of men who had existed before Adam. They were excavating in a small cave at the side of a modest hill outside the village of La Chapelle-aux-Saints in southern France. After three years of relentless digging, they had reached the cavern floor and an unnatural ditch that had been filled in during the age of European mammoths. In a grave, they came upon a skeleton of a human being, Neanderthal man. Their relentless curiosity led them to uncover the oldest known burial in the history of the world. In a reverent palsied silence they barely appreciated what they had discovered. The abbes in a transfixed ambiguity uncovered what was later accurately described by the French paleontologist, Marcellin Bovie in a classic monograph.

The burial, it is told, was undertaken by Neanderthals who appeared as monstrous fetuses of aborted pregnancies with terrifying large heads attached to thick short necks. Their faces were enormous and repulsively human. The few even shorter females that were present possessed the same brow ridges, receding chins, and foreheads. These Neanderthal humans, with their eyes fixed on a clan member lying at their feet, can be envisioned to have been in a frightful suspension. He was immobile beyond the stillness of those that observed him. He had become unresponsive, soon to be in rigor mortis. His mouth was ajar and his vapid eyes had just released a last tear that migrated downward into a pool made by the auricle of his external ear. There was a beard that would continue to grow; there were nails that would also indicate their own signs of post mortem life.

Ann Terry White has written that paleontologists, then and now, have reasoned that this Neanderthal skeleton discovered by the abbes was not just the oldest burial known. The skeleton lay on its back. Around the skull lay a row of stones, and all about the remains lay great numbers of worked flints and bits of ochre. Ample food had been placed next to the body. Several large flat fragments of the long bones of animals lay about the skeleton. Near the skull lay the foot bones of a great ox in a position to suggest that the entire foot of the animal had been placed there for food. All this evidence provided the theory that the Neanderthal brain began the comprehension of a spirit life beyond the grave. It was here that the brains of ancient humans began to defy death. It was here that the primordial stuff of religion sprang to life. Death could be managed and as time passed the release of the spirit from the body would create earthly ritualistic behavior beyond a primitive burial. In time, there would be the sacrifice of a Toltec Indian's beating heart, the spinning of prayer wheels by Buddhist priests, the singing of Gana by orthodox Catholic monks high up in the caves of Ethiopia and the fervent study of the Cabala by messianic rabbis.

Willis M. West points out that the spirit was long ago thought to hang around the body and close to the relatives of the deceased. Bodies had to be kept close at hand for the separation process to take place. Bodies were first kept in certain rooms and then buried under the floor. They were kept as part of the family for generations. All primitive worship began with family ancestors. The bodies and the spirits were still part of the family and by Neolithic times, when Stone Age man lived together in larger numbers, their home sites began to take on the appearance of mounds. They were unable to move away only up on top of basements full of departed relatives' skeletons.

The Neanderthal was not some kind of new monkey; he was an early human. He was included in the family of mankind because his brain was evolving a new visual symbolic neuron cluster that would forever separate him from lower pre-human forms. The new symbolic neurons could hold an image in the Neanderthal's brain long after the real image stopped stimulating the retinas of his eyes. These remembered images, as we have noted, were inhibited by ongoing visual stimulation during the daylight, but when darkness fell, the retained images would come up into consciousness as big as star bursts.

In REM sleep, modern humans dream with images retained in the visual association cortex of their brains. Dreams of modern man evolved from these first retained images that developed in the right hemisphere and in individuals with brain illness, these retained images became visual hallucinations occurring when the individual was wide-awake. In prehistoric times, with the evolution of those new visual neurons, the appearance of the nocturnal images was a matter of course and not associated with mental disease. Those newly evolved images in early humans likely created a simple-minded belief that there were visible spirits of real things in the real world. The images could be seen but could not be confirmed by any other sensory modality. However, they visually existed and appeared to be out there in the air. Early Stone Age people had no idea that the images were only psychic mirages in their brains.

And so it continued to be true. By medieval times, there were numerous reports of saintly visions that were considered bona fide. Visions that have been reported since are the same neurological off-spring of early man's new brain. Joseph Smith may have had the last significant religious vision in 1820, at Palmyra, New York.

With this new seeing brain, man became very different from all other animals. He would not just caress the sun-bleached bones of the departed, as East African elephants continue to do. He could define death as a spirit either within or out of the body.

Chapter 2

THE HOUSES OF GODS

WHAT HAPPENED TO HUMANS AFTER THEY GOT THEIR HANDS ON THE NOTION THAT THERE WAS A SPIRIT IN AND OUT OF THE BODY.

Salt Lake City, Utah, 1938

"Bim," as Clarmont David Kaminski was called as a boy by his father who mused about his own past and momentarily forgot he was talking to his son, "this is a good town for traveling men." Kaminski and his father were standing on the capital grounds overlooking the city. They had just completed an evening round of securing large night crawlers for the next day's fishing trip into Provo Canyon. The capital grounds at dusk were well watered and bait of the round worm type readily came up from soil burrows to avoid drowning. The backs of the father and son were turned away from a granite monument to Utah's early pioneers. Kaminski's father, wearing a shaggy herring bone suit with a vest buttoned all the way to its flared bottom, stood behind him. Worm procurement was more important than changing out of a business suit. His father's lanky legs had ample coverage with pants whose cuffs rolled out and over his shoe tops somewhat independent of the whole pant cuff style. Redundant folds also hid the heels of his oxford shoes now muddy from preparatory fishing labors. He wore a broad-brimmed fedora in vogue at the time. It added five inches to his six feet tall frame. He was of royal Mormon stock. He held one hand firmly around his son's anemic neck, almost a choke, but somewhere between that and an inhibited sign of affection of a Mormon elder for his only son. Unable to ask more about traveling men in Salt Lake City because of an Adam's apple held securely inoperable, David Kaminski would find it necessary to learn on his own much later about the women of Salt Lake City. With a bucket of worms swarming like a herring ball at their feet, they took in the metropolitan scene before them. In the distance, the Mormon Tabernacle and temple were down there to the right. The angel Moroni, in a constant state of trumpeting to all comers that this was the new Zion, was atop the highest temple spire. The angel, in furrowed robes, looked like ancient Roman statuary in fine layers of gold before the stripping by Visigoths and Franks. Father and son could see the vanishing points of the broad Parisian-like avenues named Temple and State running north and south. (The city streets with the extra width made some think Brigham Young who designed them, was the Mormon answer to France's Hausmann, who tore down slums to create big boulevards to move troupes against rebellious Parisians.)

Kaminski's father was named Lorenzo Calvin Kaminski. He was a dark complexioned Semitic looking man to Irish and Scottish second and third generation Mormons that cared to observe him. He had a Roman nose, pointed and sharp to enhance verbal combat. There were dark circles under his brown-green eyes; he had just gotten over a gastric ulcer. Gaunt is what he was, the personification of psychosomatic illness and hypochondriasis, good Mormon traits for the times. Renny, to some, Cal, to others, Kaminski's father was the oldest son of a family of two sisters and three brothers and one half-brother he was ashamed to mention most of his eighty-six years of life.

Lorenzo was born December 25, 1897, just around the time the world-famous neuroscientist Charcot died in Paris at the age of sixty-nine. His father was a Mormon bishop who oversaw the business and the tithing of the western regions of the LDS Church sprawling into the state of Idaho. He was known as the church president for that region and drove the buckboard roads in a horse drawn wagon to Burley, Twin Falls, across the Snake River by ferry to Boise, up to Mountain Home over the Stedman cut-off taken by pioneers before his time to avoid hostile Indians, up to Idaho Falls, down to Pocatello and then back to Oakley, Idaho, the family home. Lorenzo Calvin Kaminski's neurotic personality was shaped by the rigid moral demands of the old Mormon Church and the men like his own father that ran it. It was appropriately named the Church of Latter Day Saints of Jesus Christ. It was a "forme frist" of the first Roman Church of Jesus Christ, existing in a light bulb and combustion machine age with the anachronistic character of churches two thousand years older. Strangely enough, the LDS church in the 1840's was no different from any others when Mormons made their flight for reasons the Pilgrims thought were their own. In 1873, T.B.H. Stenhouse, once a Mormon himself, wrote: "The Mormon organization is thorough and complete. It permeates every position and condition of life, and controls and governs everything from the cradle to the grave. It is a combination of iron military rule and Jesuitical penetration and perseverance." Those words defined the suppressive, intolerable, and unmistakable control of not just Mormons, but of all followers of other religions.

Things had not changed in the early 1900's and it was that insufferable character of religion that gave Lorenzo Kaminski his dour personality and his gastric ulcer. For his own sanity, he felt it necessary to avoid the door of the Mormon Church from the age of seventeen and for the rest of his life.

The Mormon religion was a glimpse into the past of all new faiths on a rocky road to salvation in religious history. Like early Christian sects of the first and second centuries, Mormons did not gain social acceptance with a carte blanche. The Mormons were persecuted, thrown out of Ohio, Missouri and Illinois. They were tarred and feathered and imprisoned. Their homes and farms were burned. Men, women and even children were killed by members of the Methodist, Presbyterian and Baptist forms of Christianity. Even the militias of sovereign states of the United States of America were enjoined against them. This violent arousal was the same resentment that the "Unholy Roman Pagan Empire" felt against Jews and early Christians; the Roman Catholic Church felt when Luther posted his ninety-five theses; the Pueblo Indians felt when force-fed by Father Bartholome de las Casas in the mid sixteenth century to stomach a new religion of monotheism for polytheism, monogamy for polygamy. Piss on the katema rites. Burn the masks and costumes. Inquisitions, crusades, persecutions of Huguenots, the burning of Savonarola, one must realize that the Neanderthal brain created a powerful idea attached to deep emotions of survival not only during but after life. Over thousands of years, the spirit idea of the brain multiplied like a puree of warm yeast and brown sugar. The product spawned was fought over by its makers all along the way. What a great idea, spirit and body, what miserable stewardship! The carnage that poured out of man following this early brain invention was caused by genetic survival instruction of the ancient reptilian brain.

The instruction dictates that there must be control of those in the territory; they must be dominated. In humans, the reptilian code has spread from the physical control of individuals to their tools, i.e. their brains' newly evolved means of communication and the products of thinking and ultimately to their ideas about an after-life. The "spirit idea" is one of the oldest ideas that leaders of hierarchical human groups have used to control their members. It also is an idea that throughout history has been rammed down the throats of competitors for territory.

Before the New Testament identification of Christian religious conflicts, there were the struggles of the Babylonians, the Syrians, the Hittites and the Canaanites. The Egyptian gods of new societies were up against the previous gods of older societies. The moon god took over the sun god and ravaged his temples. The spirit idea rendered its havoc not only on the old gods and on the infidels of other religions, but also on its own members in lethal earnest. The spirit concept and its taboos so richly revealed by the early Stone Age Hawaiians paint a vivid picture. "You, peasant, step on that piece of ground the king just walked upon and you will be clubbed to death on the spot. It is taboo. Don't look at him. Bow your head. Looking at him is taboo. Get down, way down until your chin and stomach are on the ground. Your eyes must be hidden from him. Your arms must be outstretched until he passes or you get the club. He is god." (It was a Hawaiian Stone Age walk on egg shells.)

Mystic animism that came out of the original spirit idea is well chronicled by the Toynbees who tell of life in the spirit cocoon controlled by a few. Everything had a spirit and you had better watch out because the "Anti-Santa" was coming to the town of every human body. It was no Eden. There was no noble savage. Everything in nature was chiseled into the ancient mind after Neanderthal with either pacific or demonic intent. Man lived in a caldron of satanic, insufferable fear and appeasement of those spirits. It was only five hundred years ago that Incas took on the mountain sickness trek each year and sacrificed children through freezing mummification at the summits of Andean peaks. The pagan Indian mind of the New Stone Age feared to offend and needed to appease the sun god's circadian miracle. What an incredible device to control human behavior was the spirit idea that came out of a human brain development that could better remember a visual image.

Spirits within a human body during life and without the body after death, spirits in all things in nature especially in animals of prey and predation, following the same order evolved into the earliest religions best identified by the cave drawings of Cro-Magnons in the French Vezere Valley at the dawn of the Magdalenian Period. The Cro-Magnons likely worshipped the animals of prey that sustained them. Animal worship probably derived from an early animalistic human brain that was capable of very little but reflex

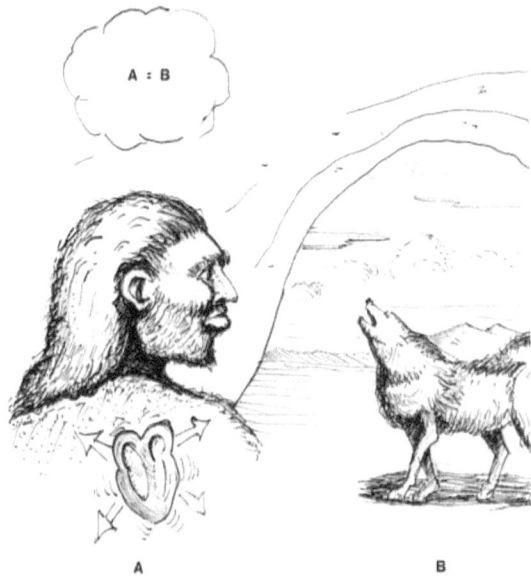

Figure (2-1) Hominid brains without symbolic language could not appreciate subjective self from external objects. By simple conditioning an internal body sensation (A) became associated with the environmental object (B). The object became as much self as the inner conscious body sensation and gave rise to external objects as spirits capable of being in or out of the body. It also explains why early man, especially Cro-Magnon drew images of themselves as part beast and part human.

conditioning. Early hunters saw an animal of prey and felt the rush of excitement within their abdomens and chests. (Something we appreciate today as an autonomic nervous system discharge in the abdominal plexus having been activated by the alarm center within the brain.) The sight of the animal and the inner sensation were imperviously mixed and in terms of spirit or simple conditioning, the animal was as much in him as it was out there in the animal. See figure 2-1. (Early Christian pictures show the devil with horns, hoofs and tail. These records demonstrate the remnants of animal worship that turned into devil form.) Animal worship was mixed in transitional Babylonian and Assyrian religions that also worshipped ancestors. The colossal alabaster man-beasts found in the Palace of Sargon, now in the Louvre, depicted the ancient belief that the spirit of man was partly the beast that sustained him. (Those sphinx-like, half-man, half-beast statues are the next of kin to the man-beast cave drawing of Trois Freres, St. Giroud, France.)

All primitive peoples worshipped their ancestors along with a belief in spirits. The beginning of Egyptian religion in 5000 B.C. also consisted of animal and ancestor worship. Each family worshipped its ancestors. Dynasty simply meant family. Egypt was ruled by families whose ancestor gods became celestial gods of those that were ruled. The depth of that rule, in the minds of the believers, would place them at work on pyramids for their god-kings for a great deal of their lives.

Greeks of 1500 B.C. continued to worship, as did the Egyptians, ancestors who became celestial bodies. They worshipped a sun god and continued to worship their ancestors, one of whom had become that sun god. The smallest unit of Greeks worshipping their ancestors was the clan, an enlarged kind of family of up to sixty individuals. Each clan elder was the priest for ancestor worship. He provided meals and magic formulas for the spirits of the departed. (The process continues in some modern Christian religions in which the head of the household blesses the meal on the table.)

Clans evolved into tribes composed of groups of clans believing in and worshipping a common ancestor. The clan elder of the leading clan was the king of the tribe and its priest. Tribes became cities and city-states. Greek religious habits became Roman, but with new pagan names. Religion and government were immutably interwoven from the beginning of their ancient history. The king was, by an ancient prehistoric idea and the logic that followed, both the lord of the land and the chief priest of its holy ghosts.

Christianity would not change that union between church and state in the Roman Empire. In a fit of atavistic hallucination reminiscent of Neanderthals' visions, Emperor Constantine converted to Christianity when the sign of the cross appeared emblazoned in the night sky accompanied by the words "in hoc signo vinces". Constantine's conversion may actually have been more pragmatic, since at that time there were two Christians to every pagan in the Roman Empire. There was to be a new state religion however, and a new theocracy, in which Constantine would still remain as the king and the chief priest. He began a new campaign that T. B. H. Stenhouse described of the early Mormons. The spirituous fanfare of pagan life was to be torn of its old clothes. Pan and Priapus and Venus were cast out of the temples. The body was sacred and should be covered. After death, the body should be buried and kept as a holy item not to be disturbed. Suppression, control, restraint of the body and spirit were the big new ideas of monotheism. With this new outfit for the body, civilized Europe entered the Dark Ages. Polytheistic good spirits (gods) were banned in a papal cremation. No more sun worship, there was to be only one heavenly body of a father. The bad spirits beat the rap, but got new names; no longer demons, they came out in fashionable terms such as "Satan" and other devils out of hell. James C. Coleman states that "Man in the first century A.D. became the battleground of the devil and God for the possession of his spirit." Man's spirit was now called a SOUL, still controlled by the priestly kings and by spirits with new names.

The spirit concept of the Old Stone Age brain trudges along with its own evolution. Religious thinking is a continuum of a brain idea that has evolved over time, much as animal species have evolved. There is the holy sacrament (sacrifice?). There are the temples of Jupiter that are changed just a bit to fit the Catholic taste. The Pantheon of Agrippa has become a Christian church. There are no idols but there are the Pieta and the ubiquitous sacred models of Christ dead on his cross. There are those Christian and Jewish medals around the necks of believers, those Greek Orthodox icons. (Did not early Christians, when in power, hammer away the unsightly genitals of pagan gods leaving them dismembered or on bishopric direction, clothing them with fig leaves? Wasn't St. Dionysus once a pagan god?) Why is it that pagan times of sacredness, the solstices and each equinox prevail but with secular names and different meanings? The finger of the original brain idea "having writ moves on" never fully purging its earlier foundations of control. What an interesting way to start thinking about the mind. For thousands of years, the mind was a spirit that didn't reside in the brain. Where was it? Sometimes in the body and sometimes downstairs in the basement coffin and then up in the stars. Time would tell.

Chapter 3

BODY OVER MIND

HOW THE BODY SCIENCES DROPPED OUT OF SPIRIT TERRITORY.

Department of Anatomy, University of Washington, School of
Medicine, 1954

There was a dank and sterile theater then, no ushers but a need for eyes
to be dark-adapted. There were no left-handed seats only right-handed
ones with a paddle-board of wood to write upon. The murmurings of
anticipation were there once the seats were occupied; then the usual hush
when the house lights rose to illuminate the stage. You could then see that
this was an amphitheater in which the audience, not in any irreverence,
looked down on the actors the way they did in Greco-Roman times. No
applause now for the solo performer about to deliver his lecture on the
autonomic nervous system. The hush turned to absolute silence.

What a stunning figure he was, dressed in white, a vicar's collar and
a white butcher's apron to match. The costume was unique for gross
anatomists, no other choices for the job. The thespian hesitated only for
a second while he made a head-nod directing his assistant to ready the
slide projector for his performance. Professor Richard Meyer Johannson,
M.D., professor and head of the Department of Anatomy needed only a
few props. One was the dissection table upon which he rested a three foot
long maple pointer with a black rubber tip; another was a white projection
screen upon which works of anatomical artists from Vesalius, Eustachio
and Vidius in the sixteenth century, to Wren, Vieussens and Gautier d'
Argoty in the seventeenth, to Frank H. Netter in the twentieth century,

would eventually be displayed. The oratory was to come in the smashing projection of a guided missile. It emanated with the noise of an air-cooled German machine gun. It bounced off the ceiling, the walls, the floor and now the tracers of his voice could be seen in the dark of night. The lights were out. You could catch momentary reflections of his athletic figure and fog gray crew cut darting in and around projected anatomical Latin words made more obscure by his Teutonic accent. This was not a lyrical version of the foot bone is connected to the ankle bone; it was Wagner.

Anatomy was war. Every man was for himself. In the bustling darkness out popped hand-held flashlights on and off like fireflies about to mate at dusk. These were prepared combatants, students who knew it was impossible to take notes in the dark. The left-handers were leaning far to the right trying to negotiate that note board on the opposite side of their cerebral inclination. Lights or no lights, this was combat. The amphitheater was just the general's briefing room where he exposed his own mastery of the artistic and diagrammatic representations of the human body.

Action would take place in the dissecting laboratory; cadavers would not be spared. Nothing can ever match the depth of indelibility of a room with twenty-five corpses on their sacrificial tables draped to form a white mountain range of anatomical relief. You could see the peaks of feet, valleys of abdomens, pelvic crests, rib cages and cranial parts to the summits of the noses.

"My God, what are you doing? You don't need a knife and fork to eat a sandwich." Medical student David Kaminski's wife of seven months objected to a fundamental break in the etiquette of eating sandwiches. She was learning her first lesson of "like father like son." Kaminski looked at his sandwich with his mouth tightly closed and its corners drawn down into a pout. He was revealing his familial neurotic nature exposed by the study of gross anatomy. With the fork and knife having created two halves of his whole wheat bread, he used the same tools to expose the contents of a now vivisected sandwich. A layer of mayonnaise, then a layer of lettuce leaf and a final layer of cold turkey breast, a kind of muscle, dead flesh. The specimen was adroitly removed.

"What in God's name are you doing now?" Kaminski had spent the morning on the battlefield of his cadaver along with three other students. That cadaver would lie at their disposal for as long as three months of probing, cutting and the teasing of tissue until the crematorium put to fire what was left of the corpse.

Anatomical dissection required dexterity and the use of carbolic acid, the embalming fluid that does its work on the living as well as the dead. Kaminski's hands would reek of carbolic acid all the days of his life in one way or another. No washing, no deodorant soap, no counter odor would remove its specific significance. The living hand tainted would set off olfactory revulsion of the experiences of the laboratory. The closer it came to the mouth and nose, the worse it became. Kaminski loaded his fork with a freshly cut section of sandwich. The offering was delivered into his mouth far enough away from his hand and the odor of death.

Professor Johannson was a "latter day saint" of the Body Church. (His kind are still worshipped to this day with endowed chairs of scientific learning.) He came from a long lineage of priests that evolved from the Neanderthal's first idea of body and a spirit. Throughout all of recorded civilization, priests as we have spoken, eventually organized spirit control into religions. The spirit idea also resulted in a priestly management of body ills. Roger Sorenson points out that early powerful priests were the healers, and are evident today as witch doctors. Priests initially were in charge of the new concept of body and spirit altogether. Spirits and body were healthy only when good spirits were in and bad spirits were out of the body. The priest had to exorcise bad spirits as shaman. The body of humans controlled by animism was, for millennia, not to be tampered with in spite of an occasional trephination of the skull. Once the spirit left the body, it had transitional tasks to perform and was needed around the house of relatives. Don't even think about finding out how it worked; what was inside; the body was not to be violated.

Ancient medical priests that eventually produced the likes of Professor Johannson were for unknown reasons splintered away from spiritual temple duties around the time of the ancient Greeks. Most early Greek physicians were more faith healers than physicians. They were poor anatomists because of spiritual beliefs about body sanctity. Then Greek healers that became physicians began to look under the skins of the dead. They were enjoying an unknown idea of free thought and action that all other early civilizations tied to a spiritual mentality forbad. Hippocrates (460-357 B.C.) took a bold step without a scalpel and denied the intervention of deities and demons in the development of disease. "For my own part, I do not believe that the human body is ever befouled by a god." It was probably this free-thinking that got Hippocrates a union of his own. As Ingles states: "Such thoughts weren't welcome in the temples."

Prior to Hippocrates, the Egyptian priests were already performing dissection in preparation for the mummification process. Although this procedure was done to preserve the body for an afterlife in the spirit world, there were men who carried their curiosity beyond what was proscribed in the priestly removal of organs. One such man was Alemaeon of Croton (570-500 B.C.), a Greek Pythagorean physician, who became the most eminent pre-Socratic embryologist we can recall. Through dissection, he discovered the optic nerve and realized that the brain was the central organ of sensation and intellectual action. These were good observations, but ones that would not be honored for another one thousand years. The temples were safe in spite of these revelations because the work of the body went on separately from the work of the spirit. For all the while, inquiries of body interest never assailed the sovereignty of the matters of spirit. The spirit basked in the light of its non-reflection and was protected for centuries. There was no habeas corpus.

Romans who continued the work of Hippocrates. Asclepiades, Aretaeus and Galen would not let the investigation of the body rest, but the spirit priests went through a changing of the guard. Christianity entered the scene. While not true of other cultures around the world with gods to worship, Europe fell into the Dark Ages following the rise of Christianity. The body sciences in this darkness lost their way as well. The Gestapo appeared at the door. ("Back in your cell. It's lock up time; the spirits are back.") The magnificence of Greco-Roman thinking about the body was out of there, back on its side of the drawn line in man's thinking about spirit and body. Demonology consequently flourished in the Middle Ages. There are some who feel that mental disorders became frequent then and that their incidence was considerably greater than in ancient times.

Madness then had peculiar qualities of prehistoric suggestibility. As Coleman states: "There was a peculiar trend in mental illness, involving the widespread occurrences of group mental disorders which were apparently mainly hysterical in nature. Whole groups of people were affected simultaneously." There were dancing manias. Tarantism resulted in epidemic raving, jumping and dancing and ended with convulsions and sometimes death. The spirit was out of control, not necessarily through the excessive control of Christian doctrines of thought, but the confusion it brought to the pagan mind. European mankind had flipped out; it had gone to Saint Vitus' dance.

By the time of the Renaissance, dissection of the body slowly became resurrected. It became an acceptable means of medical study once again. The brain was again established as an organ of the body. Curiosity was aroused as to where the main spirit of the body resided in the brain. There was great confusion about all those other spirits that came and went within the body. Medical investigators in the early Renaissance had a great difficulty in explaining body functions without using a spirit concept of action in the body. It was important for physicians to think in terms of spirits to keep the priests happy, to keep themselves out of trouble. They were all god-fearing men, those early body scientists, including one of man's greatest early scientific thinkers, Rene Descartes. In 1619, Descartes was faced with the awesome problem of explaining that the human soul was capable of scientific thought. His first contentions were that the rational soul (mind) and the human body existed independently. Keeping to the spirit-god and body separation beliefs, Descartes would reason that his soul and spirit came from god, but his senses of perception were in some way part of his body.

In *The Passions of the Soul*, Descartes presents the doctrine that the primary point of interaction between mind and body is a small, delicately suspended gland in the brain, the pineal gland. Decisions of the mind can cause the pineal gland to sway one way or the other, thus altering the course of physiological processes. The direction of the "animal spirits" or subtle fluids of physiological processes, Descartes believed to be essentially involved in human sensations and body movements. Conversely he thought that the mind responded to motions in the pineal gland* brought about by the various bodily changes involved in sensory experience and emotion. (See figure 3-1). Descartes was trying diligently to preserve the godly Christian order of things and still understand his scientific thinking mind. His utterances tell us of his struggle to understand where and what that thing in the brain called his soul was. His devout faith sustained the idea of a separate soul and blocked the real truth that the mind was part of the brain. (He is often given the credit for the original dualistic concept that mind and body are separate entities, but nothing is further from the truth.) Descartes arrived on the scene of history

---

*   The pineal gland is considered a vestigial structure in the human brain. In certain reptiles it continues to be an organ that tells the animal when it is night or day.

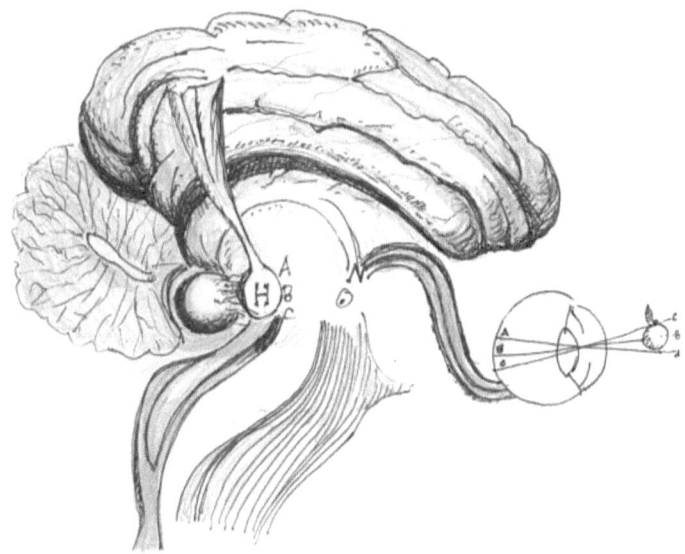

Figure (3-1) A copy of Descartes' original diagram illustrating the effect of light upon the rational soul lying in the pineal gland. From *System of Ophthalmology, The Evolution in the Eye* by Sir Stewart Duke-elder. C. V. Mosby Company, 1958.

as a deeply religious man trying to explain the rational thinking of scientific matters in terms of the thousands of years of belief that spirit-soul existed separately in or out of the body. The origin of the spirit-body dualism was Neanderthal's not his.

It was very difficult to keep spirit involved in the explanations of new scientific discoveries of body functions. Prior to Descartes, in 1543, Vesalius still proposed that food when absorbed, was endowed in the liver with a natural spirit that in the brain became animal spirit. Most early Renaissance physiologists tenaciously resisted the idea of the brain having anything to do with the spirits of the mind later to be called emotions. They maintained the old spirituous concept of affects as a function of organs outside of the brain. "The heart is slow to learn," Andrew Lloyd Weber still reminds us, and our ancestors vented their spleen when angry. Rancor and bitterness were ensconced in their livers and came forth in behavior as the gall of its bladder. The womb wandered and caused lunacy. As late as 1850, renowned Parisian physician Xavier Bichat contended emotions began in the organs of the body. This was well demonstrated in his belief that increased heart activity caused anger, and that sobbing and increased rates of respiration caused grief. Stomach distress caused resentment. Still later, in 1870, the world's first modern physiologist,

Claude Bernard, continued to embrace the idea that there was a causal effect between body fluids and physiological manifestations. When Bernard lectured at the Sorbonne on the topic of physiology of the heart, he refused to accept the belief that the heart was strictly a mechanical pump. Bernard held to the old bias that the heart caused certain emotions; the heart gave rise to an emotion of deep conviction. Thank goodness for Bernard and the persistence of thinking that our emotions were once spirits in different organs of the body. What would songwriters have done without such a notion?

In spite of being influenced by the age-old idea of spirit actions in the body, in the late nineteenth century, European scientists were working their way out of those old-fashioned notions. The process was not one without conflict however. The study of body fluids which contained spirits came to be known as the science of Vitalism in which body functions were dependent upon a special energy that was distinct from the scientific physical forces of nature. Vitalistic theory was a hybrid of the old spirit idea and new Cartesian ideas of energy.

In 1860, when Louis Pasteur established the germ theory based on the fermentation of alcohol by yeast, European science had fairly well given up Vitalistic understanding of body functions for an understanding using mathematics, physics and chemistry. Pasteur's discovery was vehemently opposed by men of science that held to a new order of chemical energy to understand body functions. Rene Dubos, in his biography of Pasteur, tells us that little by little science had expelled living forces from the domain of physiology of the body. To believe that a living thing, a microorganism, was causing fermentation and disease appeared to the major scientists of the day, Berzelius of Sweden, Liebig and Helmholtz of Germany, that Pasteur had fallen back into a retarded understanding that was vitalistic. Nonetheless, Pasteur prevailed along with other scientists who brought about a scientific systems approach to understanding the body and its organs. There were Miobus, Jackson, Koch, Virchov, Weeks, Argyle-Robertson, Lister, Bell, Golgi, Ramon y Cajal, Kolliker and many new body priests who provided new understandings of body function based on scientific investigation.

The spirit priests of nineteenth century religions were just barely in their own territory separate from that of the kings and queens, but they were still abiding to them and still providing control for them unperturbed. Body scientists now had their own territory and were of no concern to the spirit guardians as long as the body men paid their visits to the temples, paid their tithes, confessed their sins, sang the hymns, praised the individual Lord of their spirit realm.

Yet, similar to many of the storms of evolution, there came out of an unsuspected compass direction an attack on the prehistoric brain idea of a divine separation of body and soul. The idea, that gave power to the clerics, custodians of the temples of the gods, would be challenged by a member of the body sciences. The challenge would come from the study of earthworms by Charles Darwin.

Chapter 4

TERRITORIAL IMPERATIVE

HOW DARWIN CHALLENGED THE WHOLE IDEA OF A SPIRIT MIND.

"Don't tell them you go to the Mormon Church. Tell them you are a member of the Church of Latter Day Saints."

"But why, Mom, aren't they the same?"

Clarmont Kaminski was now called "David", his middle name. It didn't cause so much bullying in public schools. For his Mormon parents, from big families with limited resources, the decision to have only one child required a name for their son that would conjure up expectations of J.P. Morgan or Franz Liszt. The name "Clarmont" wasn't working in the practical world even though it stood for Fulton's monumental mark on industrial change. Thank, God, for middle names. Calling the Mormon Church the L.D.S. Church worked the same way in the ecclesiastical world of the 1930's. It was a time in American life where being a nigger or a kike or a Mormon still provoked the acts of bigotry beyond name calling. While some words are now forbidden in the culture, the name "Mormon" can still get a wry smile.

With churchly matters seemingly behind him, David Kaminski with his name revised, blended in with the offspring of the established Catholic, Protestant, and Jewish believers of the separation of spirit and body. But David's mother was going to continue to give her son instruction about the special Mormon methods of managing behavior of the herein for the hereafter. In addition to reading and writing, Mrs. Kaminski thought it best to provide the Mormon version of a religious education. The education began with a baptism down in the basement of the church, called the Stake

House. It was performed by the L.D.S. bishop in Spokane, Washington in 1940. A solemn, quiet affair, there were just the bishop, David and his attendant mother. It was a little spooky and intimidating as being led into a gas chamber by reverent deputies on Judgment Day.

"And now, in the name of the Father, the Prophet Joseph Smith, and the Twelve Apostles, I baptize you that you may take the sacrament, join the priesthood and go on a two year mission (and if you stay in line, you can pay your ten percent tithe when you become a productive man)."

Down went Kaminski's head into the chlorinated water of a hot-tub sized basin but twice as deep. His head was placed there suddenly by one of the bishop's hands and then with his other placed on Kaminski's chin, up came the head so as not to drown in the process of becoming a Latter Day Saint. The clothes of the participants having not been removed were ringing wet, but the shoes and socks placed to the side of the pool were dry.

Kaminski's old man wasn't there for the occasion nor was he present in the Stake House on any Sunday. He wasn't there with the other elders, the brothers and sisters and those in the process of acquiring those names of common ties and belief. His father didn't find a presence when it was time to pass the sacrament of bread and water that represented the flesh and blood of Jesus. What a strange atavistic act, but some of David Kaminski's Catholic buddies were following the same rites of communion but with wine and wafers. Following the long hours of Sunday's religiosity, by eleven in the morning, a young man was getting hungry and those tiny cubes of Wonder bread blessed for the occasion and washed down with a thimble of holy water tasted pretty good.

In a short time, Kaminski went to the Stake House unattended; even the maternal baptismal attendant wasn't going to church anymore. Kaminski took up the hymn book, mouthed the words and waited for the best part of the show, the giving of your testament. It wasn't easy, adults first, then the children. At the beginning, there was a long silence accompanied by coughs, squirming and gazing at the arched ceiling. Then someone, feeling the surge of the crowd mentality taking place, stood up back in the rows of believers. That someone was a she, who was shaking and tearful. She told the faithful in attendance that she was a true believer as her voice broke with sobs of joy. It spread like wildfire, the standing up and professing, but the timid would remain silently beholding with outstretched arms hanging onto the railing of the benches just ahead.

Yet things were happening to the bodies of newly baptized people like Kaminski, inside and out. Pubic hair was starting to show; nipples were taking on a new form; hips were appearing curvaceous and bodies were shooting up into adult size. Satan's urges accompanied these body changes and needed more and more expunging. Kaminski found himself fighting those satanic influences on his body; "Forgive me, God, but what am I to do with this erection?"

There were other influences on Kaminski's Mormon view of the world; the boy scouts seemed passe while a cowhide floppy baseball mitt denoted maleness. Movies and Satan's accomplices in the form of the opposite sex moved front and center. Without the constant inculcation of parents, the church and prayers for forgiveness in that once modern day of Amos and Andy and the Lone Ranger, the spirit pressured by body urges retracted back into the atmosphere from which it came.

In the dawn of civilization, the evolution of man rolled along to provide him with more of a chance at survival now that his earlier successes had produced so many more of his kind. Change was not an obvious elective alternative. Man had to change or he could not survive with so much competition. Hunting and gathering were disappearing, replaced by a more stationary society based on trade and barter, crops and commerce which resulted in higher birth rates. Coexisting with the new agrarian society were the wandering mobs and masses (the former hunters and gatherers) plundering, robbing, killing and looting. How to protect this new society from the hordes was a question that the great Roman general Marius addressed with success because of the power and organization of his Roman legions.

The world's great religions were also devised as an attempt to pacify human behavior as well as convert it with force when necessary. The religious inspirations arising out of man's more successful visual brain, however, didn't have any room for coexistence. The fundamental religions of East and West, which appeared so alienated from one another because of the crocodile nature of those doing the viewing, were actually evolution's unified mandate in action. The enlightenment the great prophets spread, by intention or not, continued the success of man awakening to less elbow room and more savages after his women. The words from the polyglot of the saints, prophets, martyrs, esthetics and monks were going to change the monkey in man's chaotic behavior.

In evolution of the brain, the great right cortex of symbolically communicating man took charge of the Orient, the great left cerebral cortex took charge of the Occident. Both hemispheric brains and their expressions in diverse cultures had it subtly in mind to curb non-survival behavior that some called man's "vegetable" nature and others called "animal". Religions' oppressive process of fettering mankind's impulses from their beginning, in odd lots and sparse distribution, to mega proportions of greater wandering populations and crowded urban environments, was eventually challenged much more successfully in the West. Because of the rise of the middle (merchant) class and the subsequent end of feudalism in the West, religious beliefs and practices, which had been "the opiate for the masses" were being questioned by this newly educated and increasingly affluent class.

Cranked up further, more change for survival was inevitable. It came as a bubo on godly behavioral modification called the scientific method. In the beginning of humanism, the sciences slept in the same bed with the religions, each enjoying their dreams separated by a bed-board of mutual understanding that science of mind and body had nothing to do with the religion of spirit and the body, until one fateful day.

By the evolutionary clock, it was a tick in time not too far from the inception of a spirituous mentality that began in a rudimentary mind. It preceded the year 1925, and Monkeyville and the Monkey Trial at Dayton, Tennessee, where William Jennings Bryan took up the gauntlet as the Spirit's advocate. He prosecuted the educator who taught scientific theory. "How dare you teach the young and innocent fatuous information that contradicts the Holy Scriptures." The Monkey Trial was a redo of an earlier script that played out the most significant modern battle between the adherents of the body spirit concept and those that began to find its faults.

There were stand-ins for the main actors, but there was no question that Charles Darwin represented the Body sciences and the Church of England represented the Spirit forces. Darwin's *Origin of the Species* was printed in 1859. It was a statement that was contrary to the holy idea of the dignity of man. It claimed that nature had not been created for man alone and that a divine power had not created mankind, but rather man had evolved from the animal world of prehistory.

Prior to Darwin's bombshell, the men of the body sciences, including those called naturalists and comparative anatomists, believed in the presence of spirit and body to the satisfaction of religion. English scientists, not unlike Bichat and Bernard of France, had spent all their lives trying to fit the round pegs of what they had studied into the square holes of religious beliefs. Those god-fearing Englishmen were especially indignant because Darwin's book was causing chaos, not only in scientific circles but in the ideas of common people who eagerly read it.

Many scientists, especially anatomists, thought Darwin's idea bombastic. One in particular, Richard Owens was considered by himself and others to be the greatest anatomist in the world. He, especially, was aroused to rage by Darwin's work. On the other hand, a rising star of anatomy, Thomas Huxley, saw his chance to contest his older rival with

Darwin's work that he championed. These stand-ins acted on behalf of the divided and confused men of science who tried to support old and contrary beliefs that persist to this day. It was "mano a mano" between two anatomical scientists, one acting on behalf of religious history, the other certainly on behalf of his career and not so certainly on behalf of science.

The world was about to turn upside down again. It was not on account of a new threatening antichrist, a new religion. It was a challenge to the theory of religion all together. The conflict was not to be fought with mail and mace, but with the civil process of gentlemanly debate. Behind Owen stood the true representative of the church, Bishop of Oxford, Samuel Wilberforce. Wilberforce was going to "smash Darwin". The dreadful solution to opposition reappeared; it was tar and feather time, once again. In the beginning the anatomist, Owen in his characteristic style, condescending and imperious at the same time, let his opponent Huxley and the audience, which became the world, know that "The human brain had certain structures which were never to be found in the brain of anthropoid apes." Unwittingly, the contestants were confused. Owen had made a good argument *for* evolution. His statement, however, was firmly opposed by Huxley. The point is the brain of man has all the structures possessed by anthropoid apes yet more, the evolved structures specific to man alone. Taking the position of imperial pagan Rome in this arena, the Bishop of Oxford had come to cast the Martyr Darwin into the jaws of the lethal beast of his reason. As history tells, this end was not achieved. The Monkey Business was not over.

Following the additional work of Darwin's student, George Romines, facial expressions in primates were found to be similar to those of humans. Therein began, unappreciated, a later startling discovery that the emotions of man's mind could be identified as being part of evolution as well. It was a beginning, but the neurological concepts of a map of the mind were flat and when you came to its edge, you fell off, back into the abyss ruled by the spirit.

Darwin's unspeakable idea that mankind was of animal origins embraced a more profound and unthinkable correlate. If it were true, then the mind, its predecessors, spirit and soul were also of animal origins. The first objections of the English clerics had to do with the apostate attack on the veracity of the Bible. By association, it included those who wrote it and from whence it came, God Himself. The logic that the brain's contents, including the mind, had an evolutionary character was not even thought of by clerics or those religion-abiding scientists. Eventually the logic would surface, but not then. Body science concerns had to do with more general body investigations of the whole species of man and his brain. Body and spirit were still separated, but with a rising discontent in some thinkers and a rejection of any disbelief by others.

Eventually scientists of the body would come to explore the idea of evolution of not just the brain, but of the mind. This exploration of the evolutionary character of the mind was done through the back door of body sciences, from the study of the mind when it slipped in to be a science. To this time in history, the mind was a philosophical and a spiritual issue. Psychology had its roots growing in mazes and experiments that did not include the human mind. It took a twist of faith to get the study of the mind away from the spirit's jurisdiction. This not so petty crime was accomplished by Sigmund Freud as he redirected the science of psychology to study the mind. The body sciences, of which psychology would be included, would eventually stumble upon the flesh of the mind.

Chapter 5

THE BODY OF EVIDENCE

HOW FREUD FOOLED THE BODY SCIENCES INTO THINKING
PSYCHOLOGY WAS ONE OF THEM.

Tremler Stern was known to his fellow classmates in medical school as "Shaky". Here was a human fizgig. Internal medical professors wondered if he had an over-active thyroid. Mind and body were revved at thirty-five thousand revolutions per minute. His pen would scribe away at examinations and for the few notes he took in class with the ferocity of a male Bowerbird preparing its nest. There were no pauses between verbal utterances; his conversations and recall of facts were a life-long sentence bound together with "ahs". While others were to take a second sip of their favorite beer, Tremler was beckoning the barman for a second and a third.

Tremler and Kaminski were good friends. Opposites attract even within the same gender. It was a pleasant relationship between the hare and the tortoise of their medical school class. Kaminski was a slow, deliberate thinker; Tremler, on the other hand, vacuumed up facts and knowledge. While his physical nature could easily be observed, it took a National Institute of Health examination about all sorts of cancer knowledge to appreciate his real genius. These examinations were given to medical students to determine if their school was getting the right material across to their students. By and large, these were examinations that all of the students felt did not tarnish the medical school's reputation, but were demanding just the same.

In a large auditorium, the examinations were handed out along with special pencils, the marks of which, automatic grading machines would recognize. Student Kaminski went on his deliberate way to answer what appeared to him a Wall of China length of multiple-choice questions. The examination required four hours for its completion. Similar to Las Vegas slot machines, the odds of multiple-choice questions were biased toward the house for slow thinkers. When the odds lengthened with questions that needed to be answered with, "all of the above, none of the above, one and two of the above", it took a long time for three cherries to come up on the machine of Kaminski's mind. Kaminski's hands began their routine perspiring. His brow became erythematous with the blotting duty of a crumpled handkerchief. It was going to be a long morning, but not for Tremler Stern. Kaminski looked up at some commotion in a distant aisle. Forty minutes had passed and Tremler could be seen moving toward an exit. "The poor son of a bitch," Kaminski thought, "he's sick." But no, Tremler had finished the exam before any other student—in one-fourth the time it took the rest of the class. The new medical school, just six years old, did not have an open grading system then. You got your papers and examinations back from their evaluation with comments, but no "A" or "C", no number like "95" or "64" out of "100". Those grades were a secret for the eyes of the faculty only. But it came to pass, that all the students in Kaminski's class intuitively knew their place and Tremler was on the very top of the academic glass mountain.

But there was a dark side to the new Dr. Stern that graduated with highest honors. He was emotionally unstable. It became evident in his internship at one of the most prestigious institutions of the country, He went from making fifty-proof beer in his basement to snitching absolute alcohol from the labs in various departments of his hospital. There were stints in recovery centers, problems with the medical disciplinary board, a divorce, loss of a medical license, drug usage and all the oblivion of not being able to cope with the stress of being a physician, father and husband. The mind is a peculiar thing; it can be so brilliant and yet so fragile and unable to manage the simple things of life. It is hard to believe the mind can be both things at the same time. Tremler's erratic history gave Kaminski hope for himself. He could live with himself a little easier after watching a genius with so much trouble. Now what did Kaminski mean? Was his "self" more than what his words described?

At the beginning of the nineteenth century, psychiatry and neurology were a combined focus of study because clinical diseases could not be easily identified as being due to a brain disease or a disease of the mind. Coming on a wave of investigation brought about by the scientific method, the birth of both psychiatric and neurologic sciences was delivered by two great pioneers, the German, Emil Kraepelin for psychiatry, and the

Frenchman, Jean Martin Charcot for neurology. Both men made use of new principles for codifying the clinical symptoms and signs of disease and then comparing them with pathological changes in the body. A disease could be established by pathological anatomical verification. To Kraepelin, we are indebted for the definition of dementia praecox, (schizophrenia) and manic-depressive psychosis. To Charcot, we have come to appreciate a great many medical conditions and illnesses, such as: the Charcot aneurysm, Charcot artery, Charcot crystalloids, Charcot Marie tooth disease, Erb-Charcot disease, Charcot fever, Charcot gait, and Charcot joint syndrome. He also identified the symptomatic differences between paralysis agitans and multiple sclerosis.

The basic identification of a disease became the modern clinical pathological conference in which a physician attending to a particular patient and treating his symptoms for a suspected illness, became more able to understand the disease of his patient. It would be the post mortem and the histopathologic examination of the patient's tissues that would establish what really happened during an illness. It was a body game that underpinned the basis of modern diagnosis and treatment.

Through this method of identifying diseases based on pathologic finding, many "mind" afflictions became "organic". For example, many dementias became wards of the body when they could be identified by specific changes in the brain. The mind diseases of syphilis, cerebral arteriosclerosis, Alzheimer, Huntington, Jakob-Creutzfeld, alcohol, uremia, pellagra and many others could be identified by changes in the brain. Charcot was puzzled by mind diseases that could not be identified by this method. Those mind diseases remained dependents of the spirit. A very common mind disorder of that time was known as an hysteria. Enter the student, Freud.

Sigmund Freud was an Austrian M.D. who had specialized in neurology. He received an appointment as lecturer on nervous diseases at the University of Vienna where he met a career-crushing obstacle. Early in his teaching career, he introduced to his physician audience a psychoneurotic (spirit disease) patient suffering from a persistent headache and mistakenly diagnosed the case as chronic localized meningitis (body disease). This mistake cost him his job and he later surfaced in Paris to study more with Charcot in 1885.

Freud's interest in hysteria, a disease that has come to be called "functional" disease can well be appreciated. The word "hysteria" today means an uncontrolled outburst of irrational emotion, fear, weeping or laughter. For the psychiatrist, then and now, it means an entirely different thing. It is a mental disorder characterized by mental dissociation leading in severe cases to multiple personality and amnesia and often to somatic symptoms such as convulsions, paralysis and sensory disturbances in the absence of "organic" disease of the nervous system.

Freud observed and treated many hysterical patients with a technique of suggestion either under hypnosis or with a new process he called "free association". Freud, a medical doctor, essentially began a new science of psychology to deal with hysterias not identified pathologically in the body. His patients received new forms of treatment based solely on verbal interaction with the doctor. Freud took one-half of Charcot's system and without pathological verification began to treat mental illness with symbolic verbal behavior. In Freud's observations of mental illness, he found characteristics of the mind that allowed him to theorize that it had parts. He carved out of the mind something new, but the term he used to describe it was old. He called it the psyche. The human personality was defined. Within it, there were the Ego, Id and Superego that have become kitchen terms of discussion.

A number of other scientists, Ivan Petrovich Pavlov and John B. Watson, being the most outstanding, also were studying behavior, but with animals. These new psychology scientists believed that the brain could be mechanically explained in terms of stimulus-response neuro-mechanisms found in animals alone. They, too, were unable to find the mind in cold and hard anatomical brain facts. Like the great American psychologist, William James, they stayed away from the mind.

Although Freud began his career as god-fearing, he renounced his faith in the Jewish religion and went so far as to hypothesize in *The Future of an Illusion* that religion in toto would eventually decay from human thinking. Among most other behavioral scientists, it was sacrilegious to challenge thousands of years of belief that the spirituous part of man was separate from his body. There was no need to identify parts of the personality in the mind.

Yet Freud was a medical doctor who successfully treated patients with mind diseases, so it was not difficult to convince his profession that his now very popular methods of taking care of patients were part of medical science. Freud's new science of psychoanalysis applied complex Germanic logic to his explanations of the mind. As he continued his clinical investigations, he realized that the mind had some peculiar characteristics that had to do with totems and taboos from man's distant past. This psyche, he had discovered and whose existence he could not prove under the microscope, would stimulate his followers to identify more of the evolutionary character of the mind. They did it under the noses of those that lived and died by the new principles of science that demanded anatomical proof.

Enter Freud's student, Jung.

Carl Gustav Jung was Freud's first, most notable student. Jung followed his reptilian evolutionary instincts and wanted his own territory. He wanted to be the primary head of the territory of the new science of psychology. He would not remain at the feet of his hierarchical master, Freud. The two separated, but Jung took the basic concepts of Freudian doctrine and modified them. This was evolution in action.

By the nineteenth century, the long process of man's struggle to understand self-identity hardly had penetrated the surface layer of the issue. Jung, still breaking ground, had ideas that began to turn the dogma of Freud away from a dichotomous understanding of self. Jung's new ideas, grounded upon Freudian principles continued to remain outside anatomical verification. For his ideas to be accepted, Jung acknowledged the ancient comprehension that the mind, the psyche, the soul, the spirit of the human are separate from the physical body. While Freud drew attention to anthropologic characteristics of the unconscious behavior of his patients, Jung appreciated there were phylogenetic aspects to that part of the psyche. Still there was no reference to where the unconscious was in the brain or where the conscious part of the psyche existed. Nothing seemed anatomically related, but Jung admitted to himself the vague appreciation that the unconscious part of the self was likely in the brain. As Ester Harding, a Jungian disciple, states: "We remain puppets of those unrecognized forces of the unconscious until consciousness is developed in relation to them." These unconscious forces are part of what Jung felt was a collective unconscious. His term prepares us for the understanding that man, the individual, must pass through what man, the species, has passed through. Hidden deep within Jung's understanding was the realization that the self must pass through the stages of development (collection) to achieve full consciousness or self-identity. Jungian thinking was on the verge of understanding the self had a genetic developmental basis. It was collective in the sense each member of the human species had basic psychic characteristics but in relative degrees. Jung's conceptualization of the mind was on the verge of saying "ontogeny recapitulates phylogeny". There was the dawn of inspirational light that the human psyche was no different in this regard than the embryos Haeckel observed in the development of the human body. Archetypes, Jung dimly conceived, were psychic manifestations of that recapitulative process that occurred in dreams, myths and legends. "We are the age-long experience of life that man and animals before him have passed." While Jung's beliefs of the psychic presence of archetypes supports a recapitulative process of phylogeny, he continued to think of them in terms of "psychic energy", not completely spiritual or physical but akin to cosmic energy of the universe. Jung compared them to crystals that were salts in solution and therefore molecules or dissociated atoms.

Continuing the evolutionary awareness of the psyche was Theodor Reik, who stated: "We cannot understand (self-identity) of an individual without insight into his development from early childhood. We cannot understand the general situation of human civilization without studying the history and the prehistory of its evolution. We have to sketch the mental and emotional prehistory of our ancestors from myths, customs, legends, and rituals." While these observations of the Freudian school acknowledged the evolutionary character of the psyche, there was no department of anatomy to empower their thinking with a body of physical evidence. Yet, evidence was mounting that the mind developed in a manner suggesting a physical process.

Two recent followers of Freud, Erich Neumann and Eric Berne, also appeared to have been sensitive to the basic dilemma of having to deal with mental diseases within the concept of a separate mind and a brain. Their evaluation of mental diseases called *functional disorders*, seemed strained in the scientific world under the burden of the old issue of pathological verification. They were aware of the scientific illegitimacy of psychiatry.

It was troublesome for Neumann and Berne not to see a mind gone wrong under a microscope. What would Virchow think of them talking about the mind that could not be identified the new scientific way? What dismay not to see the mind with microscopically silver stained nerve cells Gogli found in 1878. Not just seeking legitimacy, but likely also respecting the fathers of the body sciences and their standards of proof of disease, mind-men, especially like Neumann and Berne, started talking the body language. Neumann referred to stages of mind development as psychic organs. Mentally ill people acted as if their minds had parts that were diseased organs, he is quoted as saying. He warped an anatomical term around the mystery of the mind even though it was still a game of blind man's bluff.

Berne was fully aware of the evolutionary characteristics of the human mind, but did not know where it was in the brain. In 1961, he referred to the mind as being similar to evolutionary anatomical parts of the brain. Berne may well have felt the pressure of criticism of psychiatry to justify the use of similar anatomical terms in reference to Freudian oriented mind parts. As interest in the physical nature of the mind began to ferment in the 1960's, there might have been some embarrassment on the part of psychiatry to have such little scientific proof of the mind's objective reality. When Berne described Cobb's comment, ("The study of the emotions is now a legitimate occupation."), he provides us with the affirmation that psychiatry had arrived.

Psychiatry was likely tired of being a distant cousin of medicine. To prove the point, Berne announced his new anatomical terminology. He was no longer content with the terms: Ego, Super Ego, and Id. For public consumption he used new more understandable terms of Child, Parent and Adult. For the profession, he produced some exciting new anatomical terms: Exteropsyche, Neopsyche, and Archaeopsyche. He now regarded them as "psychic organs", structures of the mind somewhere in the brain. Without any further regard for the courtroom proof demanded by other specialties of his medical peers, Berne tells us: "The methodological problems involved in moving from organs to phenomena to substantives are not relevant to the practical applications." So back to square one, the issue remained. The substantives of Parent, Adult and Child tell us a great deal about mind behavior, but without anatomical proof. As mind and brain began their interchangeability in our thinking, it would be to the neurologists and the neurosurgeons that the proof would be forthcoming.

Chapter 6

FLESH APPEARS ON THE MIND

HOW MODERN SCIENTISTS ARE DISCOVERING THE NEURONAL
WIRING OF THE MIND.

In the early morning, Dr. Kaminski was lying in his bed somewhere between being asleep and being awake. Sprawled on a queen-sized mattress, one of Kaminski's arms was suspended over the edge of the bed and precariously hung on the edge of the night stand. Kaminski was dreaming. He remembered that. Upon being awakened by the abrupt fall of his arm from its perch on the table next to his bed, he was perplexed by the strange nature of his dream. A large baseball bat was falling toward him and he dexterously caught it at the moment he wakened to discover his arm had fallen from the table. What perplexed him came after a moment's reflection in which he pondered Freudian notions that dreams often disguised attempts to fulfill needs that were present while awake. He recalled that often he was in a dream in which he was walking to the bathroom but once standing over the toilet, his stream would not result in the emptying relief of urination. Then, when the pain got so bad, he abruptly awakened to get up and actually perform the biological need. He kept thinking that the dream was activated by an internal impulse of bladder pain signaling its fullness. The inner sensation went up to his brain which began a dream sequence of unsuccessfully urinating. Sometimes the process did not result in his awakening; it actually kept him from awakening. It was as if the dreaming brain attempted to deal with the information even though it did not have the ability to exercise the actual act of going to the bathroom and urinating. The ability to begin or to inhibit urination was somewhere in the conscious brain. Kaminski appreciated that bed wetters had not developed an adequate inhibition of the process of just dreaming and not actually urinating. In the arm incident, he reasoned, the same mental process was active. The falling arm activated a dream sequence before the jolt of the arm moving actually woke him up. In this case, the stimulus for the dream was external, not internal. The falling arm resulted in a dream that something was falling, a baseball bat. The falling arm stimulated one part of his brain before it became conscious in another. As Kaminski lay there, perplexed, he commanded himself to "get up" and "get on with the day", but nothing happened. He noted that the internal request did not cause the instantaneous result of his body moving up and out of bed. As his mind wandered a bit on other subjects, his body rose and left the bed as if it did so on its own, outside of the volition of his internal verbal command. Then he appreciated that body movements could be separate from imperative commands of the self from within, that they were not automatically united in an action. Now he could understand why so many people on the internet were inquiring about 5-hydroxy histamine because they were suffering from sleep paralysis. (In this condition, an individual's mind is awake, but his body won't move.) Thus he knew that a great deal of his body's motor actions were hooked up to his mind by neurotransmitters and that human behavior, outside of dreams, could be on-going without the individual knowing about it. Was there a brain explanation of unconscious mental behavior that Jung called the "shadow"?

The astounding findings of Freud, Jung and their followers have brought to our attention that the mind of man has an evolutionary past. Those observations have been recorded by the science of psychology and the documentation is impressive from a deductive perspective. Yet the evidence for such an assertion in terms of the kind of anatomical verification that Charcot required to establish a brain disease as being organic rather than functional, has been lacking. There has been little anatomical proof of the mind's existence in the brain. For many hundreds of years, mind was considered separate from the body. It was a part of the spirit and needed no anatomical verification. While Freudian study of the mind took a course away from spiritual control and made it a body science, psychology still paid its dues to the spirit because the mind persisted in being studied outside of anatomical scrutiny. Throughout recorded history, the study of psychology has always been in terms of mind and body. Initially within this context, it was a pre-Christian Greek philosophical conflict of two theoretical understandings of the mind and its ideational capabilities. Did ideas and thoughts come from the experiences of the body senses, i.e. from the brain or were they innately present in the appendage of the soul, the mind? With the advent of Judeo-Christian theology, an intensification of this dialectic occurred which explained human behavior as a function of the mind within the soul's domain. As Eric Klinger states in *Structure and Function of Fantasy*, "Two long-run consequences of the patristic psychology were, first, the incorporation of all psychological functions into the construct of soul, in which they were divorced from material bodily processes and insulated from objective observation; and, second, the postulation of a free, causeless will that played a role in all activity, including ideation . . . outside the realm of objective natural-scientific explanation." However, the scientific method began to loosen the foundation stones of the seemingly indestructible concept that the mind was separate from the body.

In Freud's day, medical science began its earnest remodeling of spirit concepts. Vitalism theories, remnants of the spirit model of explanation, were just beginning to be discarded and verification by scientific means of pathologic identification was emerging. Following Charcot, men like Virchow, Koch and Pasteur were demonstrating anatomical evidence of disease in the brain without a spirit concept. This identification was not to be the case for diseases of the mind beyond the classification that Charcot brought to them. Mind was still too much a part of the soul and the spirit of man. It was an extremely difficult ideational stronghold to break down.

Scientific psychological investigation in modern times had two probing heads. One studied animals, such as white rats, and made generalizations about human behavior based on these animal models. The other got tied up in Freudian explanations of human behavior based on evolutionary theories of the mind, what we appreciate as psychoanalysis and the medical field of psychiatry. Since Freud begot a medical legitimacy for the study of the mind, it has gone down an apparent blind alley until modern psychiatry fell out of love with unverifiable Freudian dogma. Psychiatry, based on Freudian theory, was discovering that it was very difficult to talk patients out of their mental diseases, no matter how long the analysis took.

Psychiatry, a purely medical discipline today, has very little to do with psychology of the past, especially those ideas about an evolutionary mind. Modern psychiatry is deeply involved in the treatment of mental diseases from the far side of the body territory. Psychiatry is managed from a body point of view within the isolationism and complexity of biochemical neurotransmitters. Diagnostic criteria for mind diseases have been markedly redefined away from behavioral characteristics. While psychiatry and psychology go their own ways other sciences have moved toward unifying mind and brain.

Neurology and the neurosurgical sciences began in the early 1930's to appreciate certain cortical structures of the brain, when injured or surgically removed, resulted in drastic changes in the human mind. Neurologists began to understand some of the more evolved aspects of the human mind had a neural basis. It was a messy business that was embarrassing to both neurology and psychiatry. Neurology was wandering into psychiatric territory. Nonetheless, a number of neuroscientists, Hebb, Penfield, Moniz, Lima and Brickner demonstrated that reasoning and decision making, things that for centuries were attributed to the immaterial mind and its will, were seriously altered when damage to the cerebral cortices of the frontal lobes had occurred. Damage to these brain structures resulted in regressive human behavior of dependency and personality changes that were socially inappropriate.

In the 1970's, a Darwinian follower uncovered anatomical evidence of man's evolutionary brain that would put some meat on the skinny unification of mind and brain. The man who reawakened scientific thinking about an evolutionary mind that could be verified anatomically was Paul D. MacLean, Chief of Brain Evolution and Behavior at the National Institute of Mental Health in Bethesda, Maryland. MacLean brought to our attention that we humans have a mind of three basic evolutionary components that can be identified structurally and histochemically in the brain. MacLean took the giant leap of Darwinian faith and placed scientific evidence for that faith on the table for verifiable scrutiny. He convincingly demonstrated human brain behavior has evolved from simian brain behavior; behavior we have heretofore considered a legacy of the mind. As an example, male squirrel monkeys utilize an aggressive genital display in an attempt to dominate other males. The visual display is a fully erect penis. This display is often associated with grinding of the teeth. Both penile erection and bruxism have been observed in man during periods of REM sleep indicating a suppressed behavior of the past. The penile display is similar to aggressive reptile behavior that is the same in courtship or in the show of aggression to rivals. This behavior has been derived from specific brain structures found in old mammals and reptiles; structures also found in the human brain. With an evolutionary prospective, one can trace this animal behavior to man. "Pan, Priapus, Amon, Min and others are all historically associated with fertility and often portrayed with an enlarged or erect phallus that is superstitiously endowed with the power of protection. In Asia Minor, for example, phallic images associated with Priapus were placed at vantage points for the protection of orchards. In primitive cultures in different parts of the world, the territorial aggressive implications of penile display are illustrated by house guard-stone monuments showing an erect phallus—used to mark territorial boundaries." Gajdusek, in a 1970 paper on Stone Age man, called attention to the parallel between the display behavior of squirrel monkeys and certain behavior of Melanesian tribes in which penile display is characteristic for expressing aggression and dominance. MacLean concludes that primitive man evolved to cover his genitals not from modesty, but to reduce the social tensions that genital display would produce. The naked man who flashes from the backdrop of his raincoat, regressively displays in a pathologic state of mind what once had more strategic functions.

The three animal evolutionary components described by MacLean are the basic components of the mind of the human species. MacLean, in his extensive reports and lectures, began to use the terms, mind and brain interchangeably. The components of the human self, Reptilian, Paleomammalian and Neomammalian, undergo recapitulation in each individual's mind as it matures either partially or completely in modern society. The basic evolutionary chasse of the mind presented by MacLean can be verified anatomically. The mind is being transformed from untouchable spirit to touchable brain.

In contrast to our primitive mind elements, the contemporary neurologist, Antonio R. Damasio draws our attention to a neural basis for the most highly evolved element of the human mind located in the frontal lobes. In his study of Phineas Gage, who had a classic injury to the frontal regions of the brain, and in his analysis of diseases and injuries of a similar nature in others, Damasio identified general psychiatric changes in all the subjects. These patients suffered from bouts of rage, an absence of empathy, a lack of embarrassment, inexplicable sadness, and an inability to make choices and act on them. These changes occurred separately from any damage to things we call intelligence or memory.

Damasio makes the most important point that is hoped for in the understanding of the mind. There is a difference between mind and brain, but the truth is, the mind is an anatomical part of the brain. Until the last half of the twentieth century, no medical science has been inclined to find out where in the brain the mind is located. Listen to Damasio's insight that gets to the root of the problem.

"The distinction between diseases of brain and mind, between neurological problems and psychological or psychiatric ones, is an unfortunate cultural inheritance that permeates society and medicine. It reflects a basic ignorance of the relation between brain and mind. Diseases of the brain are seen as tragedies visited on people who cannot be blamed for their condition while diseases of the mind, especially those that affect conduct and emotion, are seen as social inconveniences for which sufferers have much to answer. Individuals are to be blamed for their character flaws, defective emotional modulation . . . such as lack of willpower . . ." This insight of a new anatomical reality of disease of the mind touches upon an even more significant paradigm. A normal mind is not a blessing granted at birth to every human but like the whole brain, the mind must develop along with the brain.

As we have seen the idea of a separate mind and brain is as old as the species of mankind. The concept will not go down easily. Until there is an understanding that the mind with its evolutionary roots must properly develop anew in each newborn human, we will build more prisons, pursue solutions of social inequality with more inept programs, and attempt to cure mind diseases with addictive chemicals and unrealistic short term remedies. The point is further accentuated by recent declarations of Alyson McCain, a child psychologist at Warwick, R.I. and Stewart Gordon, a pediatrician at Louisiana State University Health Sciences Center. They have observed that much mind development can be observed in PET scans of children's brains. Children who have suffered neglect and abuse at certain critical times of mind development, develop fear, wariness and other mind abnormalities that don't go away no matter how nice things get thereafter. These observations point out the reality of a hardwired mind that develops in fixed periods of time.

The mind, after the investigations of Damasio, MacLean, Penfield and others, is finding an anatomical home in the brain. On the one hand, Damasio has identified the neural basis for the highest level of human mind evolution in the frontal lobes. His findings are based on case studies of individuals whose thought processes were altered by injuries to the frontal lobes. MacLean, on the other hand, has begun to identify the older animal aspects of the mind's evolutionary elements in the brain. These scientists, while finding anatomical parts of the mind in the brain, are examining the tail and head of the mind without fully appreciating that they are working on the *same mind*. The recognition of highly developed, hardwired mind functions and their anatomical location have not been fully connected to deeper more primitive aspects of human mind function and anatomy. There is a great terra incognito of the mind between those boundaries. It is not so much unknown, but not plotted on the proper map. The prehistoric and historic evolution of the Hominid portion of the human mind documented by Wilber and others, has not been placed in a sequence between man's modern highest mind sense of self and the ancient history of his self-identity from the dim past of other animal species.

In the beginning of a shift in our thinking, the mind creates a theory, and with our current scientific tools, theories become objective facts.

The theory that the mind is really a part of the brain will require another time-bound, labored step through the evolutionary process to become an objective fact. When there is finally a complete acceptance that the mind is a part of the brain, the next fact that must be established is that the mind is the thinking self.

PART III

Introduction

Human self-identity has evolved over an unfathomable period of time from a single cell sense of self, to small aquatic multi-celled animals with a rudimentary nervous system, and then to a self-identity that included a body made up of cells. Further evolution resulted in a reptilian brain sense of self that would include not just a body-self but a territorial sense of self. Continued evolution resulted in a still larger nervous system that created a self in which old mammalian and simian behavior modified the reptile's solipsistic territorial and hierarchical self-identity to include other members of the same species.

Evolution of the genus that included hominids brought forth a nervous system that extended and simultaneously began to deplete the reptilian, old mammalian and simian core of self-identity with first greater visual memory and visual communication and then greater auditory memory and auditory communication. The most sophisticated human self-identity has evolved through a process of auditory and visual internal-communication we call thinking. Thinking has given the human the ability to create ideas of a symbolic nature that for the most part turn into physical realities, thereby expanding self-identity into cosmic proportions.

When a human is born, he or she rapidly develops self-identity in a staged process that recapitulates the long evolutionary history of human self-identity. This process is know as ontogeny. Ontogenetic development of human self-identity is not an automatic or strictly a genetically inherited process. We appreciate great variations in intelligence and personalities of humans and, in the recent past, those differences were ascribed only to germ plasma variations that were present at the very beginning of an individual's life.

In contrast to strict genetic determinism, this theory of self-identity that includes the mind, proscribes that mind-self-identity is dependent upon developmental stages that require external stimulation from other humans within a fixed time frame. Without these staged external inputs, defective self-identity results. The mind, as part of self-identity, can become defective in an absence of proper external stimulation and the self becomes stunted. The stunting we call psychopathology reflects older stages of human self-identity.

The developmental process of achieving maximum self-identity can best be evaluated by the contemporary science of ECOLOGICAL-DEVELOPMENTAL BIOLOGY, the study of the integration of environmental and genetic forces that result in the observable attributes of species. Eco-Devo biology has the basic assumption that organisms with the same genes can turn out differently depending on the environment in which the developing organism finds itself. Attention must be jarred into appreciating the environment is not just territory, but also the humans in it. In the development of a human, other humans around are as much his or her environment as the climate is. The science of Eco-Devo biology also provides the assumption that the specific environmental differences provide a process of "genetic assimilation" in which external or environmental "switches" trigger genetic variations of development. In full self-identity development, there are stages in which this triggering process must be activated by other humans.

The process is readily understood from the work of Dusheck who points out that ostriches are born with calluses on their legs. While calluses are easily understood to be an environmental effect on skin, they appear at birth, before the environment has any chance to bring them about. This is an example of genetic assimilation in which the external stimulus has over time changed the phenotypic structure of the ostrich. Contrary to the recent past belief that random mutations are the only reason changes in an animal's phenotype occur, the Eco-Devo science provides a reinvestment into the early observations of evolution that theorized environment was just as important as genes in determining the final outcome of an organism.

This appears to be the case in human development where environmental human triggering mechanisms are necessary to bring about full development of a growing human. Sensory neurons with the genetic potential for development of brain components initially must be stimulated before they can become internally assimilated. First, the infant's sensory brain neurons must be stimulated from a parent's motor neurons before the child can develop its own internal sensory-motor activities of mind. This need is clear as we observe auditory symbolic language development in the infant. Without the stimulation of language capabilities of the human mind, the mind develops without the ability to communicate not just with others, but also with itself in the process of thinking. There are many varieties of thinking; some are very primitive and must be discarded for more modern forms. It all requires triggering; what we simply think of as training and education.

An unusual example of a triggering anomaly occurred when a young mother began, for reasons she felt were to her child's advantage, to use only sign language to communicate with the child early in its development. As the child grew it refused or was unable to speak except by the process of signing. The mother unwittingly had created a child that was essentially retarded with respect to verbal communication.

Parenting is an awesome responsibility in the development of the human mind. The wasting of a human mind can occur long before it is recognized. Unfortunately, the right to give birth and the rights of parenthood have been viewed as inalienable elements of human behavior. In our modern society, these rights should be exercised only after the potential parents are fully aware of and accept responsibility for the requirements of rearing a child to achieve a full human self-identity.

Chapter 1

Pre-birth Ontogeny

How the cellular and the humeral sense of self develops.

Both grandfathers of David Kaminski's children died in their hospital beds after suffering cerebral strokes. The old men had lived to the ripe age of eighty-six, but died a year apart. The last five years of their lives were isolated and lonely. Both lapsed into a slow senile depression when their mates of over fifty years preceded them in death. Visits to octogenarians in their hospital deathbeds were spooky and distasteful for family members aware of the inevitable. For relatives that were physicians, the institutions that handled the transition between illness and the hereafter brought mixed feelings. To them, hospitals had been familiar second homes, but the constant tug on the emotions associated with death and illness gave them reason to want to return to the first ones.

There were four generations of physicians on the maternal side of the Kaminski family. When Almar Orensten, M.D., the oldest member was about to die, one family visitor to his sick bed was his daughter, Doctor Barbara. She had practiced medicine with her father thirty of the fifty years the patriarch physician had served. Gathered around his deathbed, those that loved him had a lot of anger as well as sadness.

"Damn it," one thought, "why are you doing this to us, Granddad?"

Dr. Orensten's surviving family, including three grandchildren, was standing at his bedside muted by the gravity of his illness. Then, Dr. Barbara pulled up the bed sheet and revealed an ancient foot whose big toe looked as surprised as a field mouse exposed in a once hidden burrow.

Dr. Barbara took the exposed foot and tickled its plantar surface. There was a slow upward movement of the big toe. Then she forcefully twisted that big toe and nothing happened as she watched in earnest. His leg did not withdraw nor did his face show any sign of pain.

"God, Barbara," her sister, Mrs. Kaminski exclaimed, "how can you be so cruel?"

No reply came from Dr. Barbara. The family filed out into the hospital corridor.

"Why did you try to hurt Granddad, Auntie?" the youngest grand kid asked.

Dr. Barbara sat him down as the others continued on. She took out of her purse a loose-leaf notebook and a pen and drew a line diagram of the spinal column.

"You see, Kimball, (this child was named after one of the first Mormon apostles), this is a spinal reflex. You tickle the foot here and a message is sent to the spinal cord and there a message is sent back down the leg to that big toe and tells it to move."

"Yeah, but why did you pinch it so hard?"

"Well," she said, as she continued to draw lines up into an oval blob representing the brain, "when you pinch the toe real hard, so it causes pain, that message does not go just to the spinal cord and back out again, it goes up the lower part of the brain where the pain center is located. That part of Granddad's brain didn't do what it was supposed to do. Nothing happened to him. He should have made a violent jerky movement to get his toe away from that pain. You see, I wasn't trying to hurt Granddad. I wanted to know what part of his brain was still working. Kimball, Granddad is only alive below that part of his brain that responds to pain. He is just a little bit alive."

We have accepted the premise that self-identity has many manifestations depending upon the degree of animal complexity. Self-identity is what a particular organism considers self, which is separate from non-self. It is a way of defining the many existing life forms. Life can be simple as in the single cell or very complex as in the human animal. As Ray Bradbury says we humans are the "watchers" of the animal kingdom. We are the only life form that is conscious that other life forms have a self-identity. In all other animals, there is not consciousness other than its own limited self-identity. The German zoologist, Jakob J. von Uexkull in his principal work of 1926, *Theoretical Biology*, made the point very clearly as he suggested that each animal no matter how small or complex lives in a world of its own, an "Umwelt", an enclosing world or own world which surrounds each creature. The "Umwelt" consists of only those objects in the outer world to which its sensory organs allow it to respond. Von Uexkull discovered that living organisms respond only to stimuli that produce in it either an efferent or an afferent impulse, that is, the animal responds to stimuli that produce either an impulse to action or a sense impression. He describes the world of a wood tick to make his point.

"At a certain stage of its life cycle the wood tick needs the blood of a warm-blooded animal for reproduction. It climbs onto a twig or blade of grass and goes into a dormant state until a warm-blooded animal passes its perch, the smell of the animal's sweat makes it let go of its hold on the twig and drop into the beast so that it can feast on its blood." Von Uexkull gathered a number of ticks in the dormant state and kept them in his laboratory where they remained entirely inactive until he put a drop of the acid which gives sweat its characteristic odor near them. They then promptly came to life and went through their whole cycle of movement. "One tick was seventeen years dormant, but upon smelling sweat acid, came to life."

The Umwelt or state of consciousness of the wood tick is obviously very limited in contrast to humans. Von Uexkull was a Darwinian thinker. He confirms the insight that each progressively more complex animal and each stage of human development has a self-awareness, a limited identity about what exists. The human has the self-identity of all the animal species to some degree packed in its nervous system, but those early senses of self don't register in our conscious minds. There really is a *sub* conscious to our awareness that goes back to the beginning of life itself.

Developing in the womb, the infant has no idea who it is, but its cellular and humoral micro immune system does. Like the wood tick, self-identity is marginally limited during human development inside the womb. At this stage of human life, the Umwelt is a world limited to a cellular self and serum that protect against predators of microscopic size. The territorial world of the infant's body is connected to the blood supply of its mother who provides some of that limited self-identity. Immune serum derived from the mother provides the unborn infant with a self-identity of a most primitive humeral degree. This serum and newly emerging T and B lymphocytic cells of the fetus become the infant's transplacental micro immunity, his micro self-identity. In utero, this is the only self-identity of a human infant. Human consciousness of self is limited just to immune cells and serum that can identify self from non-self. The mother provides the fetus with many antibodies developed by her own immune system against antigens to which she has become immune.

When the mother's own immune system fails to recognize the infant as completely her own there can be big problems. This occurs when the mother's immune system partially rejects the fetus as in Rh factor isoimmunization in which maternal antibodies attack the infant's red blood cells and create hemolysis and other serious consequences for the infant's nervous system.

In the ontogenetic development of a newborn child the immune cells and serum change in such a way that they become part of a greater system of self-identities that include the human mind. Before birth, however, the immune cellular and humoral stage of ontogenetic development recapitulates the human species phylogenetic evolution. It is an echo of evolution in which single amoeba-like cells became symbiotically joined to coelenterates that had just developed an inner layer of cells that started to secrete toxins against predators.

The primitive stage of human self-identity that is present before birth does not just join with the developing nervous system but continues to develop on its own through a great part of an individual's life time. This is a primary example of lateral associated development of a human self-identity component. Early self-identity components continue to mature, but that maturation is modulated by newer developing components that bind older parts to the control of newer ones.

The primary immune sense of self has been thought of as autonomous. We don't have any control of its functions. This is a long-standing conception regarding the micro-immune system. It is not readily appreciated that it is under the control of the autonomic nervous system. (In a similar earlier scientific awareness, the visceral nervous system that takes care of the inner organs was called autonomic because it first was thought to be outside of conscious, willful control of the mind. It seemed to have a life of its own like the micro immune system.) However, contemporary investigation has uncovered a chain of control of these early self-identity systems by the central nervous system and its mind. Because humans are not conscious of the activities of these early systems in their own bodies, we consider them as subconscious. They are in us, but acting without our conscious awareness. That concept is now being challenged. By acquiring auditory symbolic knowledge of their presence, humans can become conscious of their presence and influence their actions. Today, such an example of the process of a mind's influencing immunity is being established in the new science of "psycho-neuro-immunology".

Chapter 2

THE REPTILIAN STAGE OF HUMAN ONTOGENY

HOW THE BASE EMOTIONS DEVELOP.

Dr. Kaminski and his eccentric friend, the psychiatrist, Quigley, often got together to wonder where the mind was in the brain. These two men would often peel the onionskins of their discussions into the wee hours of binge drinking on vacations and professional out-of-town meetings. On one such occasion, the men had retired from the rigors of administering to native Mexicans in the Sonora desert. They went there with other physicians, dentists and paramedical help by private aircraft flown out of Long Beach and Santa Monica, California. They were part of an organization that called themselves the "Flying Samaritans". Doing good for Mexican peasants in the 1970's and 80's was very much mixed up in their minds with taking relief from the rigors of the highly competitive American practice of medicine.

On one occasion, after attending to patients in a Sonora pueblo called Testarazo, Dr. Quigley told a chilling story about one of those minds they were trying to understand.

"Honest ta God, David, I can't remember her name. It's been a few years, but I'll never forget what she confided that day. She came to me as a new patient, obviously agitated, but in a stony detached way, almost some kind of emotional denial that made me see how grave things were for her." Quigley sucked on his Pacifico beer as if an antidote made necessary by the medicinal jolt of a shot of Tequila. Swallowing quickly he continued his story.

"I think her name was Bridgeman, whatever, the way she told her bizarre story, and I was supposed to help her. Jesus Christ, after hearing it, I needed help myself."

Mrs. Bridgeman told her therapist that she had been driving to work during a sudden blizzard and her car went out of control and got stuck on the shoulder of the highway. The next thing she remembered, a car slammed into the rear of her car without injuring her. The man driving the other car got out and the two exchanged driver's license numbers and insurance companies. The man strongly protested a fault in the matter because the lady's car was projecting into the highway and had made a sudden un-signaled move to get there. Time passed and the man's insurance company stood behind him and refused to pay for the damages to Mrs. Bridgeman's car. Not known to the institutions like insurance companies was the cloaked domestic fact that Mrs. Bridgeman was the only butterfly in an avid husband's collection. Mr. Bridgeman, in his avocation and in his own mind, was the "godfather" and "hit man" for the Mafia in the protection of his wife. For many weeks, Quigley was told, Mr. Bridgeman, a city policeman who loved to tinker with cars, ranted and raved at the accident's outcome, a mistrial of justice, a crime against his innocent possession. Months continued to pass and on one occasion, Mrs. Bridgeman read in the local newspaper, quite by chance, that the gentleman that had struck her car had died in a terrible accident near Grant's Pass, Oregon. He died in a car mishap in which his van plummeted down a steep embankment in the Siskiyou Mountains. The cause, the paper reported, was an unsuspected failure of the brake line. Still weeks later, she also read without perturbation that a local insurance company's building had burned to the ground. It didn't seem out of the ordinary even when she realized it was the same insurance company that had refused to reimburse her for damages to her car during that stormy night. Still much later, standing before his wife in a mood of accomplished vengeance, intoxicated with self-righteousness, Mr. Bridgeman leaned down with his face close to his wife's trained and obliging ear and proclaimed, "Baby, do you have any idea how much I love you? Those sons-of-bitches had it coming."

Wanting an internal explanation, Quigley finished his beer asking, "How did that cop end up with a mind that was fashionable during the Dark Ages?"

Prior to birth, the infant has been provided with a fundamental cellular immune sense of self that continues to develop long afterwards. Birth, however, brings forth the first monumental brain structure that further defines a human living organism as separate from an alien world. Anoxia announces to the newborn that it must breathe or die. The process is involuntary; a reflex genetically established for all creatures dependent upon oxygen to survive. It's not a superficial kind of disturbance, but a searing pain of the most primitive kind that signals actual tissue destruction. At birth, self-identity becomes a function of a most primitive awareness of the neural signal of tissue death—pain. We are in this exacting moment essentially an organism that interprets self as either pacific or in the process of dying. This process takes place in the brain stem. It is here in the lower reaches of the brain, the primitive self emerges with its pain-limited awareness. The body pain sense of self is mediated by special identity nerve cells of two distinct developing systems of neurons, the autonomic and the somato-sensory component of the central nervous system. The former brings to consciousness pain coming from structures inside the body, from organs that include the heart, bowel, and the stomach. The latter brings to consciousness pain coming from the surface of the body and from joints and muscles. The autonomic nervous system is in a process of joining to the central nervous system, as the immune system is joining to the autonomic nervous system. Each new system of developing self-identity joins to a more complex component that will control it and thereby inhibit its freedom of action.

It is an appropriate moment to examine the rudimentary anatomy and special neuro-physiology of the reptilian component of the human brain for the understanding of its role in self-identity.

It can be spoken of as the nuclear core of the brain's expression of human self-identity and our primary emotions. Below the reptilian nuclear component of identity neurons is the part of the brain called the "brain stem" within which most of our special sensory neurons join to become part of the brain. The reptilian center positions itself as the seed from which roots descend into the earth for sensory nourishment and from which the brain ascends into a trunk, limbs and foliage of its neo-cortex. (See figure 2-1).

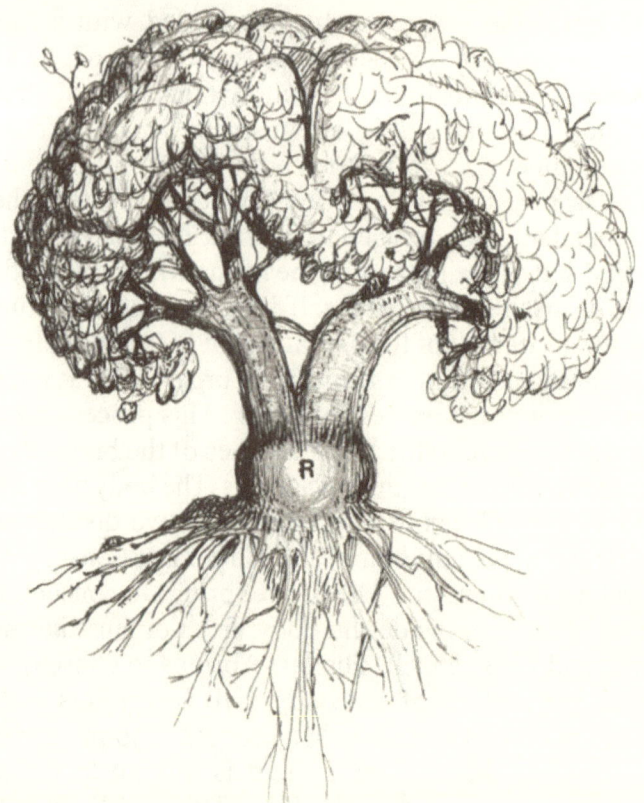

Figure (2-1): The tree of self-identity emanates from the core of neurons (R) within the reptilian component of self-identity.

The reptilian analog of the human brain has been most recently identified by MacLean in his description of the *triune brain* of man. In the reptilian component of the triune brain, he includes certain brain structures of the mid-brain called the Corpus Striatum, (the Caudate nucleus and the Putamen) and the Globus Pallidus. These structures historically have been considered to play only a motor function role for animal behavior. It became MacLean's contention that they actually provided the basic reptilian behavior of defending territory, hunting, mating and forming social hierarchies. It must further be appreciated that the reptilian brain element provides the human emotions of fear and anger associated with the behavior of flight or fight. Therefore, the reptilian analog not only consists of those structures proposed by MacLean, but also the hypothalamus and a primitive cortical element of the paleopallium or old brain. This cortical element, called the amygdala, has been previously considered to be part of the rhinencephalon or that part of the more evolved brain characteristic of paleomammals. But it is more reasonable to include it as part of the reptilian component because of the experiments that reveal its function.

The basic emotions of fear and anger states of reptilian consciousness in humans have been elucidated by experiments in which destruction of the amygdalae and the piriform areas adjacent to them eliminates fear and anger responses in mammals and renders them pacific and hyper-sexual, while stimulation of the amygdalae results in aggressive and violent forms of sexual behavior. Other experiments that stimulate the dorso medial nucleus of the hypothalamus result in rage. Similarly, destruction of the ventral medial nucleus of the hypothalamus also produces rage.

As pointed out by MacLean, the brain of reptiles and paleomammals, as well as early simian species, demonstrate fighting is a significant element in mating. One has only to observe a cat in heat to appreciate this association. MacLean's work on squirrel monkeys confirms the reptilian component's neural basis of erect genital display in both aggressive encounters with other males and attempts at copulation with females.

From these data, it readily can be appreciated that man's reptilian behavior for survival against competitors and in sexual acts of reproduction are violent acts. It is this behavior of reptiles and early mammals that must be successfully modulated in human development as it recapitulates the phylogenetic history of our primitive ancestors. From the understanding of the need for an appropriate recapitulative modification of reptilian behavior, children who are inhibited from developing a normal reptilian expression of competition, those who remain fearful and inhibited, often retain hyper-sexuality. Violent sex crimes become all the more understandable.

As evolution produced mammals, this ancient brain of reptiles became joined to the evolved mammalian brain. This combination of aggressive-pacific behavior of the two brain elements found in mammals was again modified in neomammals and still further in human brains. This evolutionary history of controlling aggression must be successfully negotiated in a delicate drama of recapitulation during individual human brain development.

Erich Fromm in *The Anatomy of Human Destructiveness* identifies human aggression as having two basic forms. One is an appropriate genetically provided defense of self and species within a territory that all animals possess. The other he defines as an inappropriate use of cruelty against our own kind. The model does not show that the genetic appropriate form of aggression is more than defensive. The reptile and most other animals also demonstrate the essential simplistic form of aggression against one's own kind in maintaining hierarchical dominance of its members.

There is a long history, an actual evolutionary struggle, of different cultures of mankind to survive by being aggressive against outsiders and insiders. With increasing complexity of the brain in human evolution, there has also been a greater complexity of both aggression and the means to contain it. We are still deeply involved in the struggle. There was the claw and now the hydrogen bomb. What Fromm feels is inappropriate or abnormal aggression continues to be the norm of less pacific cultures. He is correct to call sadistic, masochistic and necrophilic forms of aggression against humans as inappropriate for modern pacific cultures. Yet, in human history, they were the norm and are still practiced as a standard in some cultures today. Let's take a look at the acceptance of mid-eastern forms of aggression against those inside and those outside of Iraq, for example. Let's look further to the cruel and unusual punishment and the suspension of human rights (granted by the constitution) that have occurred in our own culture because of war.

Fromm makes a case for evolution because of his concern regarding "abnormal aggression". What may be labeled "abnormal" in a pacific society is in reality a look into man's past history. The socialization of man is but a thin veneer, and when challenged by a threat to self, that society regresses to its original, hostile, war-like, reptilian world. Fromm's psychoanalytical explanation of abnormal aggression is based on the defective containment of older, bombastic childhood aggression, which brings us back to mother and infant.

At two weeks, the infant's brain begins a significant increase in the complexity of self-identity with the activation of the primitive reptilian sense of self. At this time, the infant acquires a taste sense of reality characteristic of reptiles. This newly developing reptilian brain component later is identified around several months of age when an infant is noted to put everything it can get its hands on in its mouth. This stage of development has been previously appreciated as an oral stage of development that follows an earlier sucking reflexive behavior. The attention of psychology has been focused on the motor aspect of the infant's behavior. While not inaccurate, the sensory aspect of these primitive oral actions is not fully appreciated. Tasting is a reptilian process and demonstrates the nature of codifying taste sensations in the now active early developing reptilian cortical memories of how things taste. Paleomammals that evolved after this primitive sensory awareness, use a different sense in their reality testing; they smell first before they taste anything that goes into their mouths.

The infant brain quickly acquires a taste sensation of its mother's milk. The process of acquiring the gustatory reptilian sense of self takes the infant beyond a sense of body destructive pain and its cellular immune self. As we recall, the chief sense of the reptilian nervous system is taste provided by a forked tongue that senses its primary world, its Umwelt, in the form of complex molecular energies often associated with heat. This newly developing stage of human self-identity brings about an appreciation by the infant of a new sense of self that involves the presence or absence of an out of body sensation which is the taste of its mother's milk. The child becomes aware of the milk taste but not the presence of a mother that provides it.

Reptilian self-identity development initiated by taste in the infant soon brings about two magnificent improvements for its survival. This brain component now starting to develop in the lower brain, provides the human with the conscious emotional awareness of FEAR and ANGER. These first important human emotions forewarn of impending pain and eventual tissue destruction. The newly born infant, now aware of its mother's milk with gustatory sensory awareness, experiences the absence of that milk with a new consciousness of fear and anger, not pain. This new stage of reptilian neuronal self-identity takes place near the hypothalamus and surrounding structures called the "R-complex" by MacLean. In a two week-old infant, this new sense of being is identified by the visible behavior of primitive fear and anger in fits of crying associated with episodes of hunger. At five to seven months of age, the infant is characterized by a further development of this brain component when the infant is observed to be afraid of every new external sound and sight, especially when they emanate from a human stranger. The child can only find comfort in the arms of its mother.

The presence of the mother first inhibits pain from internal sources, such as hunger, and then from external sources such as adverse temperature, pressure and position. She initiates the infant's development of its own reptilian brain component. She begins the transition from pain appreciation to the appreciation of impending pain with a new state of consciousness—fear. She will in succession, next inhibit the child's new sense of self that anticipates pain with fear.

In her maternal role, we have only seen a loving caring parent. We have not seen that in so providing, she actually is stimulating a primitive brain component that establishes a mature human with an ancient reptilian form of survival. To become human, the component must be modified with additional stimulation from another fundamental lower brain element, the limbic system that in turn inhibits the component of the reptile. In the mother's role of inhibition, she provides an external brain that simulates the development of the child's own new brain components that will perform her tasks. Neurobiologists call the process "entraining". It involves stimulating sensory neurons of the infant with the motor neurons of the mother.

In this newly developing brain component of the reptile, the neural structures of body maintenance occur. Control begins of blood pressure, water excretion and water balance of the body. Control of temperature, appetite and sleep develop. The hypothalamus of the R—complex develops a greater control of the autonomic nervous system and in turn, the micro immune system. While these functions have been elaborated by science, until recently, there has been scant information about the effect of the R-complex on human behavior. This reptilian system of the brain also results in the mature human expressions of fear of pain and responses to it with anger. Fear and anger emotions appear to have little to do with the early maternal function of entraining an infant to acquire them. Yet, human development reveals the imperfect process when the development is less than human.

In an attempt to understand reptilian brain development, let us propose a preposterous experiment. We inject a toxin into a infant's brain that stops further vertical human brain development, but it does not interfere with initial development of the analog of a reptile's brain. Upward growth of other stages of brain development become checked by the toxin. What might we expect to see in an adult after such an experiment? There would be a human with a body of a human, but the neurological self-identity of a reptile. There would be an individual who would view the world from only a strict prospective of avoiding pain with its senses of fear and anger and its responses of flight or fight. An individual would develop with a sense of self that includes only those basic emotions and would remain animal-like unable to appreciate music, art, or any other joys of human experience. He would appreciate all other humans as threatening predators. He would be driven by a compulsive need to control a fixed territory and a hierarchy of rivals and mates. Love would not exist in any form. The subject would have a human pain-aware body sense of self and an immune system. He would defend his territory out of a fear that it was his own body. This human would be inhuman.

While this experiment appears preposterous, the process is going on in human development every day. A perturbing number of individuals in our modern western culture fail to develop normally at this level of self-identity, for reasons we will later explore. While they have achieved some semblance of human behavior that makes them appear human and because they can be seen to have a human body in human clothing, they are really atavistic throwbacks to a prior prehistoric sense of self-identity. Their primitive minds keep them fearful, in the shadows of society. They have a bonehead easily provoked reptilian reality. They exist as men did thousands of years ago with a bare control of their animal tendencies of kill or be killed. Contemporary habitual criminals are examples of that unimaginable experiment. We don't need any more experimental evidence. What makes habitual criminals obscure from a prospective of mind development is complexly three-fold. While they have an early defective R-complex development that provides them with killer mentalities, they continue to have a meager vertical mind development that provides them with a limited language capability. This language capability is defective in that lying is an impaired way of thinking. They are pathologically dualistic in as much as they do not develop a firm neurological joining of the auditory symbolic language cortex with the visual-motor cortex. Their right and left brain hemispheres are not unified in a civilized development. Most of their sense of self is pre-human, expressing behavior we consider criminal. Furthermore, society has not appreciated that socio and psychopathic illness does not have to do with free will and the ability to make decisions of right or wrong. Psychopathic individuals cannot be blamed for a character that will not be altered by severe punishment. How many more millions of people will be incarcerated before it is understood that the problem can only be fixed by bringing about a proper childhood development of this evolutionary part of the brain?

Mind development requires specific human stimulation to achieve normality. As we previously have shown in the evolution of language, there are external auditory steps of stimulation from human sources that activate sensory language cortical neurons of brains that have not yet acquired but are capable of language. At lower stages of human development prior to language, a similar circumstance is required to develop properly the normal pre-language emotional natures. A child must rely on its mother's immune system to start his own. A child must be stimulated by its mother to calm body signals of pain. The infant requires maternal stimulation to develop its reptilian brain component properly. She is necessary to start the process with her milk and she is necessary to calm sensations of fear and anger of body pain and of strangers. The reptilian component must be modulated through a lengthy period of childhood development. From the calming of fear of strangers at five to seven months, the infant must be led through a reptilian development while other mind development comes into play. The mother first provides calming with sensory input to the infant for pain and fear of pain from body sources and then from objects in the environment. This is done with somatic sensory input of appropriate degrees of temperature, pressure, sound and light as well as taste and smell. When the child accesses simian development and is capable of recognizing the facial and auditory expressions of calm, the mother must be present to stimulate the child with those facial expressions one of which we call a smile. Parents must be available to modify socially a child's first reptilian destructive urges at age eighteen to twenty-four months. Cats get choked; vases are pushed onto the floor; siblings are smothered in their cribs; parents' faces are scratched; and eyes are the object a child's poking finger. After guiding a child through its early fears, it must be guided through the aggressive impulses of this brain component. The parent must then be present to teach the child to stick up for itself against the aggression of others. The child must be taught to be wary of the influence of groups at a simian stage of development. These groups might attempt to enlist the immature child to participate first, in visual mimicry and then, in language induced antisocial behavior. The teacher must be present to provide problem solving techniques for the child or adolescent in his interpersonal relationships without the use of physical violence, without put-downs or insults of verbal cruelty and control. The child must be taught to avoid subtle reptilian behavior we have come to call ego behavior. He must be taught to negotiate solutions with others, not to withdraw in flight or fight in emotional bouts of anger, sulking and pouting.

The role of the parent can be appreciated as a critical pivot in the mind's development. Parenting must not be taken lightly. It cannot allow children to pass into adulthood in a thoughtless rite of passage provided by an unchecked flow of hormones. Parenting will paint the character of a culture whose leadership must insist on its civilized nature. Western culture, unfortunately, is passing through a rather violent reactionary departure from old suppressive religious values about sex. We see the transition in the unbridled nature of sexual profligacy in all of the entertainment medias. Even though sexual behavior appears to signify freedom and is not necessary for developing territorial and economic expansion, it needs cultural guidance. It is not what it used to be in the year 100 A.D. It now has a character within modern society beyond that of just the begetting of children, but it still needs control. It is far past a time of sparse human populations in which large families were believed to insure the survival of the species. Tribal societies in Africa, including somewhat modern Kenya, still hold to the belief that a family is more assured of economic security with a greater number of sons in individual families. China takes the opposite view in its drudgery of over-population by limiting families to one child. Parenting, whether it is one child or many children, holds in its hands the early fate of what a child's mind will become, how, for example, the child will fit into his society and reflect the standards of his particular culture.

What self-identity becomes with the initiation of its reptilian component is especially important to the ills of society. A child should not be raised entirely by a television set, an older sister or a paid au pair. Absentee parenting at this stage of early mind development is too costly; the price of failure is too high. As Arthur Koestler points out in *Astride the Two Cultures*, by the age of fourteen, the average child will have witnessed eighteen thousand murders on television. If one of those average children has had a defective modulation of its maturing reptilian brain, his disturbed responses to violence in his living room will bring about mass murders of school children and teachers in epidemic form. Racial and ethnic elements of modern society that are associated with extreme degrees of sociopathic behavior have not been given the opportunity to learn how to be parents. It is the cultural obligation to give them that opportunity. Those that have been given the opportunity must return to the obligations of parenting.

In the management of a developing child, parenting is required to walk a narrow line between abandonment and over-control. There is a delicate parental knowledge that must be exercised to inhibit an out-of-control reptilian development. Two well-appreciated rearing problems that work their way into adult mental illness and dissatisfaction outside of criminality are fear of abandonment and its opposite, fear of over-control. Problems from abandonment can obviously lead to criminal behavior, but there are also mental problems less than criminal that are the result of abandonment. Relative degrees of abandonment can leave an adult unable to cope without another person or the company of others; he can't find happiness unless he is holding hands or at a cocktail party. Excessive control of a child is a problem as much as abandonment in some poorly developed families when a child-parent with an unbridled reptilian brain component remains at home and ruthlessly punishes a child. Such circumstances have led to physical and mental abuse of the child as well as death from too zealous "discipline".

Over-control is caused by a parent who lacks knowledge that there is a timetable for letting a child go on its own, to make mistakes within a safe framework of reason. Over-control can lead to a child who is unable to think independently or to be alone. The adult so inclined remains in a state of fear of acting alone without someone's permission. He hardly appreciates the independence of self-reliance. He is prone to drug abuse to alleviate his fears of being alone. Without appropriate parenting, the savage in man will return to dominate the culture. That ignoble savage is unleashed by a dysfunctional improperly developed reptilian mind. When children raise children, they beget children who become soft, pliable dependent drones of a culture, or psycho and social anomalies but still dependent on culture.

The Umwelt of the reptile is rigid hierarchical control of a territory. Through evolution this fundamental basis for survival changes in other species that inhibit the original formula, but don't entirely rid themselves of it. So we see basic behavior in mammals and humans that reveal the reptile's character, but it becomes difficult to identify unless we have the original formula in mind. Alfred Korzybski, in *Science and Sanity*, likens the reptilian reality to a crude map of what the world is. These maps are varied in each individual, but the basic map of the world is genetically provided by the reptilian formula that variously expresses its character through incomplete modification in early development and lifetime experiences. When you look closely it can be seen to have driven mankind into endless compulsive hierarchical behavior. This mentality has corrupted every aspect of human brain development. Hardly any usable idea has not been distorted by this basic animal behavior that needs to control.

A hierarchy is most easily demonstrated by the flagrant pecking order in chickens. It is apparent in the behavior of lions and seals. It can be identified throughout man's history. Robert E. Alberti and Michael Emmons, in *Your Perfect Right* discuss the role of the hierarchy in humans. "All of mankind evaluates human beings on scales which make some persons better than others." In their review, the authors find that adults perceive themselves to be better than children; bosses are senior to employees; men are superior women; Whites are higher up than Blacks; physicians are more worthy than plumbers, and so on. The authors see hierarchical behavior creates all our social and inter-personal problems due to this need for dominance. The evidence is exhausting. Geographically, land is divided into territories called countries, each, without exception, consists of members struggling and fighting in a workable dominance system of government to preserve boundaries. Politically, there is a constant historical and contemporary need to dominate other people via wars, assimilation and conquest of one geographic area by another. Internal territorial conflicts all have been achieved by taking power with a hierarchical political system. Religiously, regardless of the type or ideal, there is a need in all monotheistic belief systems to organize as a hierarchy. Indeed, the principal use of the word hierarchy has a clerical origin. Economically, business in its highest expression, the corporation, presents itself with the pyramidal configuration of the hierarchy. Let us not omit mention of the military, however, which represents the most spectacular organization of a hierarchy. Socially, our western organizations, from country clubs, professional groups, labor unions to street gangs, all demonstrate the dominance theme with their exclusion and privacy. The Hindu beliefs bring to scale the fullest expression of this socio-religious issue in the caste system that allows the Untouchable to be hopeful in the next life of rising to a better social position.

Modified, evolved reptilian behavior is so automatic in humans that it goes on without our being aware that we are acting in a simple drama of hierarchical dominance. What makes this element of human behavior difficult to understand and recognize is the behavior is cloaked in a number of clever social disguises. Most difficult to expose is dominance behavior between two individuals. Language most often clouds the dominance scheme. A matter of likes and dislikes and the acceptance or rejection of limited reality models that are different for two individuals result in conflicts as to which one is *right*. "Might is right" has an evolutionary origin and who is *right* is going to turn out to be dominant, the one who decides, and the one who is more able to impale his *right* on another's *right*. "Right" often backs down to primitive behavior of the reptile with sulking silence, withdrawal, anger, rejection and even violence. Marriage conflicts and all the fall-out of those conflicts—alienation, divorce, affairs, and assault come from this single diluted reptilian survival formula. The time has come for it to be recognized as an ancient element of human brains and for evolution to continue to modify peacefully its genetic presence.

Chapter 3

THE OLD MAMMALIAN STAGE
OF HUMAN ONTOGENY

HOW THE LIMBIC SYSTEM OF THE BRAIN DEVELOPS.

David Kaminski's parents were brought up to embrace the Mormon religion. Although his parents gave up the orthodox practice of that religion in adult life, they were profoundly influenced by its doctrines. Mormonism was a modern old testamentary way of life in the 1930's. There was a simple order to things, God, Father, Mother, children. It was a heavenly and earthly hierarchy to live by. The order left women as chattel and children not to be seen or heard unless they were echoes and images of the Holy Scriptures. Kaminski's parents endured a childhood within a family patriarchy that would make Abraham proud. On his way to becoming a patriarch, Kaminski's father found it hard to trust women, trust them to bend to his ways. He insisted on subservience and proof they upheld the saintly behavior of female chastity. As he explored the realm of the opposite sex for a suitable candidate, he used a Cinderella shoe-fitting technique to guide him. The moral imperative that was later put in his son's library of proper attitudes about sex was a simple one: "If she lets you do it, then she has let some other man do it." His field trials were legion in the pursuit of a holy woman. When he was thirty-five years old, he thought he had found pay dirt when he came upon a Mormon girl of eighteen, who would become his child bride. The marriage was a Pygmalion story with a twist of authoritarian control. The young bride put up with the abuses of husbandly power for many years of her life.

She was not allowed to forget the order of things in a Christian marriage. Kaminski's father was the supreme power over his wife. He even changed her given name. His need for control of his mate had no limits. Not unlike another legend, he became threatened by his own son. It was a reference to an unappreciated Oedipal fear[1] with strong reptilian overtones. There was not just fear of his wife's disobedience, but still deeper down, there was fear the child was an unconscious rival. David Kaminski came into his family unable to be fully nurtured by his mother. She feared her husband and could not display her love to her child. Kaminski would become a loner and he would feel isolated for most of his life. It took years not to be intimidated by older men and to look straight into their eyes. When he was eight years of age, Kaminski even felt lonely in his own room. He was denied the parental bed when nightmares interrupted sleep. Kaminski was not just lonely but fearful of being alone especially at night and in the early morning hours. In a perceived isolation, he found a friend that would salve his loneliness. It was his penis. Indo-Chinese mothers calmed their infant children in an acceptable practice of fellatio and Freud considered masturbation a natural rite of manly transition. In the late 1800's and early 1900's, it was the devil's work as abnormal as a menstrual period.[2] Kaminski would start the process in a simple way. With words spoken only to himself, he directed a visual scene to transpire. A beautiful, adolescent priestess would appear and she was told to expose her private body and perform sexual things. Rub-a-dub-dub went his hand on the penis until the desired effect occurred in his mind, but without the release of spermatozoa. One such lonely morning, the father unexpectedly appeared and thrust aside the covers of the child's x-rated theater. His father took him by a firm grip of his scalp almost headlong down into the basement where a horse's whip was taken from a storeroom wall.

"If I ever ketch you doing that again, you're going to get ten lashes."

It was a believable possibility to a young child watching the blur of a leather loop moving violently back and forth in front of his nose. Kaminski was made to sleep with his guardian father for six months to prevent further "self-abuse". It made him sexually timid for the rest of

---

[1] In Greek mythology, Oedipus unknowingly kills his own father, King Laius of Thebes and later marries his own mother, Queen Jocasta. Such a myth can be seen as the basis of a father's fear of a son as a rival just as well as a son's appreciation of the father being a rival.

[2] In 1870, Dr. Albert King, professor of medicine at Columbian University in Washington D.C. claimed menstrual bleeding was something pathological. According to King, women's natural state was pregnancy. *The Body Project*, Joan Brumberg, Random House, 1997

his life. His father was as ignorant as others of his time, who scolded that masturbating hands would grow scales and result in other calamities. Little did those fathers know that children who must masturbate are quieting their reptilian fears with a new limbic tool, the stimulation of a pacific part of the emotional brain on a more primitive fearful one.

The limbic brain component of human self-identity is a legacy of old mammalian evolution. It is characterized by Joseph Le Doux as "the emotional brain" yet we appreciate the emotion to which he refers has two core components. The limbic one under discussion is separate from our more sinister emotional nature of reptilian fear and anger. This brain component is the discovery of French neuroscientist Paul Broca in 1878. This part of a mammal's brain prompted Darwin to study and compare human and mammalian expressions of its functions. "After Darwin there could be little doubt that humans express emotions by motor and muscular mechanism that have evolved out of similar mechanisms present in ancestral forms and exemplified in present-day vertebrates."

While the neurobiologist Shepard, in 1994, draws no attention to MacLean's work from 1976, regarding the reptilian origins of basic fear and anger emotions, he presents supporting data that vertebrates, such as reptiles, and even lower invertebrates express behaviors of hostility. So many experimental studies of emotions have been performed on mammals that the expression of fear and anger has been believed to be typical of them, not of reptiles. While it is typical for mammals, it is a derivation of reptilian brain function. From an anatomical perspective, the intimate relationship of brain structures of the Rhinencephalon, the brain of old mammals, to the hypothalamus and thalamus makes separation of emotional functions of reptiles and old mammals difficult. Nonetheless, the hypothalamus can be considered part of the R-complex or reptilian brain component of the human. It is here that rage, visceral functions of mating, courtship and hormonal regulation of typical reptilian behavior take place. It is in the reptilian component of the human brain, specifically the hypothalamus, that the autonomic nervous system gains activation with responses of fight or flight.

To best identify ontogenetic developmental factors in the human, it is imperative to assign flight and fight behavior and the emotions of fear and anger to specific brain evolution prior to the evolution of other emotions of just the opposite character. We return to MacLean to reassert the importance of the reptile in this regard. "At all events, lizards and other reptiles provide illustrations of complex prototypical patterns of behavior commonly seen in mammals, including man. In contrast to reptiles, the R-complex of mammals has been subjected to extensive investigation.

Curiously enough, however, one hundred-fifty years of experimentation have revealed remarkably little about its functions." This last comment by MacLean apparently refers to the understanding that while a great deal has been learned after one hundred-fifty years of experimentation on mammalian emotions and behavior none of it was ascribed to the reptilian component of the mammal's brain.

Old mammals blocked certain aspects of orthodox reptilian behavior. The evolved old mammalian brain inhibited its own reptilian need to fight offspring, rivals and mates. It inhibited simple emotions or expressions of actions that were lethal and based on fear of pain to the body from predators, rivals and potential mates.

New emotions came out of the evolution of the limbic brain that allowed mammals to join together as companions in love and war and in the raising of the young. These new emotions were associated with the breakdown of autocracy, a lethal sense of omnipotence. These emotions were quieting, loving and allowed for a sense of being with others in a family grouping. They did not replace reptilian egocentricity but modified it. (All reptilian values are maintained but modified and, therefore, are difficult to appreciate as separate from old mammalian character.)

MacLean demonstrates by the clinical observations of patients with seizures in the limbic system that this system alters the reptilian emotional code of solipsistic survival. The subjects in this study experienced feelings of depersonalization, eureka-type feelings, ecstatic, free-floating distortions of perception in which feelings of individuality and personal identity were lost. These are normally experienced in "petit mort" sensations of sexual orgasm and abnormally expressed in drug effects on limbic brain structures.

It is to the mother that the developing infant must reach for external stimulation of the limbic brain component. While the mother must first initiate development of the reptilian component of the child's brain and guide it through the perils of a lengthy human development, she must also start the great inhibition of that primitive reptilian survival system by the limbic system. The mother first quiets body pain of the infant, early emotional fears of body pain and then she must provide the infant with the stimulation of its limbic emotions of love and bonding with others. That bonding becomes recognizable to our observations most clearly with the response of the child at its simian or neo mammalian stage of brain development. It occurs with the recognition of a smile before the age of two. Prior to being able to recognize a visual pattern of a face, limbic bonding starts with the smell of the mother, her specific odor, no different than the smell of the mother's teat that drives the marsupial newborn to crawl from the birth canal through a forest of fur to feed. Limbic input from the mother quiets a new reptilian sense of self. As soon as the child reaches this stage of development and senses fear, limbic stimulation counters with a mother's pressure and warmth. Visual bonding with first any face and then a mother's face teaches the child how to respond with new emotions typical of old mammals that live in a temporary family kingdom of peace.

The limbic input by mother and then father in the human goes on to bring an independent internal neural inhibition of reptilian killer instincts. The limbic development of a child initiated first by parents must then be internalized independently to thwart sociopathic reptilian tendencies of its brain. The child must learn empathy, forgiveness, the giving of self to others beyond acts of aggressive sexual intimacy. It must be taught to pass through that great moment in ancient history when the victor slowly puts his club down and allows the vanquished victim at his feet to survive. The mental process that checked death in the coliseum by pagan Romans is still in transition. It is an amnesty conquered enemies of Persian kings could never imagine. Today, it often is still ignored in violent cultural unrest.

From this part of the emotional brain, humans have acquired the parental instinct, more precisely for women, the maternal instinct. Observed initially in children is their enchantment with something furry and then with the teddy bear. For girls of one year or so, it becomes symbolic play with dolls. It goes on from dolls to younger siblings that can be seen as the wards of preteen-age girls that allow the young to hang on their hips and to lock arms around care-takers' necks as human appendages.

For some, child-like parenting becomes a way of life. Restricted and stunted in the role of a child pretending to be a parent, these individuals often become bossy and controlling or whining and sulking with their children as well as their spouses. Not appreciating the role of the parent is to bring about independence, some individuals create offspring that remain dependent in their adult lives. The unfortunate consequences of an immature parenting also appear flagrantly in marriage. One partner remains the child and the other is a child playing the part of a parent as Eric Berne has pointed out. Applicable to either gender, this process is more often an issue with the female who has a deeper parenting nature. Karen Horney describes the situation well as a "tyranny of shoulds". One partner never seems to know what the other knows best.

Having a guiding source of social reference from an all-powerful parent, first mother and then father, is important in early limbic childhood development. This is a transitory input to the limbic nervous system of children. It is necessary for normal emotional child development. Every individual must pass through authoritarian parental direction before it can acquire its own authority. Military academies live by such an understanding; you must learn to take commands in order to give them. Adult interaction in marriage requires a more developed system of parenting that involves negotiation, not heated emotional one-sided decision-making about what should be in the household management of behavior.

Aside from modern conventions of society to embrace bisexuality, homosexuality and lesbianism, is it still possible to understand human sexual development within the concept of normal parenting to achieve what has been considered normal heterosexuality? This parenting includes a pacific and nurturing achievement of complete limbic development in the recapitulation of how we become and remain emotionally attracted to the opposite sex.

The process has a lengthy evolution that preoccupied Freud, many of his followers and scientists today. Aberrations don't just include gender rejection, but more subtle forms which involve parenting and marital bonding. In this regard, shining out as beacons of interest to Freud were the problems of incest and the relationship of children to their parents. It is this subject that continues to be foremost in our recollection of Freudian theory. While greatly disputed in psychiatric study today, revisionist dogma should not preclude the contribution of Freud's early attempts to understand sexuality. His observations about parent and child relationships, his theories about incest fit into an evolutionary schema of mammalian brain pacifism inhibiting reptilian brain instinctual behavior regarding reproduction.

To start from the beginning, survival of animals was not just a process of maintaining self from non-self as individual organisms in a hostile food chain of events, but also one in which an organism, due to energy depletion and entropy, made the process of reproduction just as important. Sexuality in its inception most likely began as a hostile act in which the single cellular sense of self required appreciation of organic matter either to resist being prey or to recognize prey. Self could be perpetuated by an essentially immune mechanism that this process represented. In the beginning of cellular life, smaller than cellular life forms, such as viruses, when ingested by a host cell broke down the cell's DNA and incorporated that DNA as part of their own survival needs in a process of cellular homicide. Eventually in evolution, some cells were ingested (or invaded) by other larger cells. The new process involved the splitting or sharing of DNA, not at the expense of the host cell or the invader, but the host and invader changed into another single celled organism with

121

DNA characteristics of both former cells. (This obviously is the process of sperm-egg fertilization in which self maintains self as a compromise of genes. It would seem we still are deeply involved in such a simple evolutionary process, survival without destruction of all parties.) Sharing of DNA was a major evolutionary change in survival of cells in which DNA replication changed to meiosis rather than mitosis. The act of survival of self went from replication to reproduction. It appears that it was the first sexual activity in which foreignness was accepted as self at the molecular level.

Early invertebrates continued to have the same persistent problems of survival against multi-celled animals of other genera and other invertebrate species. They needed to protect their individual multi-cellular selves and continue to reproduce. These more complex forms of life from early pre-invertebrate copulating forms to the invertebrates and mammals needed a systemic inhibitory mechanism to allow for the original process of cellular mutually non-destructive reproduction.

Therefore, the reptile's evolution as an animal appears significant as the next important process of inhibiting the self/non-self survival strategy of reproduction because with its evolution of special sensory systems, it acquired a sense of self that was territorial. A self/non-self concept of survival in a territory evolved even against the same species within that territory. One's own kind became aggressors for food and mates. Consequently, a mechanism was needed to inhibit the process of foreignness now attached to the same species in order not to destroy them. The hierarchy became the solution. The hierarchy became a fragile sharing of the territory and an additional early marginal inhibition of the self/non-self doctrine of survival. This is where Darwin was crystal clear: survival of the fittest was a mandate of not survival, per se, but of the ability to procreate on its behalf within the same species utilizing a hierarchy.

The neuro-mechanism of inhibition against same species antagonists preceded the reptile for certain. It began in less evolved animals as territorial-hierarchical survival expanded. However, reptiles are appreciated as the most significant land animal with special senses to include territory and a hierarchy as a method of survival. As it is understood, the concept of territory became a reality when the special senses projected the organism sense of self beyond its body.

In evolution, with the advent of the reptile, the inhibition of aggression during mating and against same species competitors for mating and prey within a fixed territory became more established. In a watery environment, before the reptile, the inhibitory signals to same species antagonists for prey or sex were humoral. On land, the signs were initially chemical then neuro-hormonal and eventually evolved to a distributed neuron system within the brains of animals.

The mating inhibition of foreignness of the same species was only for a short period in fish and reptiles and became more extensive in mammals that required a longer time to raise offspring even with marsupial pouches that short circuit internal gestation. Therefore, in early mammals, hormone driven mating was a process that inhibited primary survival behavior of self-against-non-self of the same species in a given territory. The inhibition evolved from a soluble chemical sensory system in early invertebrates to an air or ground borne chemical sense in reptiles to a smell system control in early mammals. Finally, the inhibitory mechanism evolved to a combination of all three in the mature neuro-hormonal and CNS distributed neuron system in humans.

The monumental evolutionary process of intra-species inhibition of aggression during copulation and for the rearing of the young is marked as an epochal change characteristic of mammals. In mammals, the rhinencephalon (limbic brain system) has evolved to provide a greater inhibition of a former short-tempered sense of a fleeting union among reptiles. It is this evolved distributed brain system of neuronal suppression of self/non-self that makes kinship possible. In old mammals, the sensory system of smell and the neuro-mechanisms associated with smell in the rhinencephalon define who is self and who is to be included as self. Males mark territory with specific smells regarding species, sex, sexual maturity and social rank. Females mark within the territory with specific smells when they are willing to engage in non-self behavior, i.e. being ready for a peaceful period of mating, the state of being in heat. After giving birth, when female mammals eventually smell their offspring as near maturation, the offspring are sensed as opponents in the territorial competitive sense. They are treated as foreign and out they go. The maturing smell of the offspring turns off brain hormone mediated inhibition of aggressive behavior. With the departure of offspring, however, the mature females shortly go back into heat that turns on an inhibition of aggressive behavior toward males again. The uriniferous marker of females tells the males the females are ready to copulate and will not act aggressively toward them. (Early female mammals were either in heat, pregnant or raising their young according to seasonal cycles best for reproduction.) The urine of the female in early estrus with its chemical inhibitor of aggressiveness toward the male also activates the process of male to male aggressiveness in "rut" behavior just prior to actual mating. The evolution of same species hierarchical behavior among males and females and the temporary inhibition of aggression between the sexes began with reptiles as a brain mechanism, but is best appreciated in mammals in the limbic brain.

The mammalian cycle is likely an elaboration of the reptilian mechanism beyond the short chemical sensory process that is characteristic of reptilian mating. Through evolution, the mammal has acquired a new larger brain on top of its reptilian brain to provide for the more extensive behavior of prolonged mating and rearing of the young. This extended non-aggressive rearing behavior appears to be an innate neurological releasing mechanism as described by Tinbergen in 1951.

Similar to the mammalian neuro-component that lessens aggression during mating and the rearing of offspring, there appears to be an innate neurological limbic brain mechanism that inhibits incest in mammals other than man. Here again self-identity in which the self is maintained from non-self is apparently manifest. With the appearance of species, self-identity went from the cell membrane, to territory, and then to like members of a given species. (Brown squirrels tolerate other brown squirrels in their environment but not black squirrels that are considered territorial foreign invaders.)

A moment of reflection might be important with respect to incest to appreciate the term "species". The word "species" brings to mind animals of a similar phenotype, similar physical characteristics that make them uniquely identifiable from others. To get a species in nature or the farm yard, it requires a selective inbreeding to acquire those unique physical characteristics. In the beginning, then, we can speculate that as species evolved, incest and inbreeding were necessary to contribute to the establishment of specific characteristics and traits which become genetic markers of a species. However, when species flourished in number, the tendency toward incest or inbreeding is observably diminished to the point of non-existence in the natural environment. Incest is in the human past as much as it has been for any other member of the animal world that we come to recognize as species specific. In all other mammals besides man, the innate neuronal inhibition of incest is quite automatic, a hereditary function of their "smell brain". In man, however, the process is more complex and must be learned. The older mammalian precursors of incest inhibition don't come automatically to man because he has lost to a great extent his ability to smell his offspring as if they were himself.

What can be ascribed to a genetic brain mechanism of incest inhibition in animals besides man accompanies the brain mechanism that provides bonding between siblings and parents. We observe many examples of a mutual sense of self-identity in a co-operative process of hunting, rearing of the young and mating in various species. The Orca species are interesting examples of nuclear families which remain together their entire lives. The male offspring stay with their mothers as members of an aquatic matriarchy, but are inhibited from copulating with them because of a more complex brain system of inhibition which may have evolved because of the long gestation period of the whale. The female's lack of more frequent cycles of estrus would allow male offspring to retain a longer non-sexual bond with their mothers, i.e. a mother-male offspring extended kinship.

In all old mammals, kinship is a non-aggressive behavior associated with reproduction, raising and protecting the young, hunting prey and defending against predators. The process is seen in earlier forms of animals, but with hardly the degree of sophistication that is found in mammals. Both mammalian females and males with offspring do not sense foreignness about each other or their offspring due to the *smell* mediated neuro-inhibition of foreignness that provides a reciprocal state, oneness with offspring and a set behavior pattern of amicability. In fish and reptiles, self/non-self mechanisms of inhibition are chemical-taste initiated. In simians, there are additional visual mechanisms. In humans, the self/non-self inhibitors are mostly auditory and visual with traces of the past sensory awareness of taste and smell.

By genetic hormonal-neural mechanisms lower mammals maintain kinship and have no incest because they sense the offspring as the same as themselves, as nothing foreign. Humans, however, are dependent upon visual and auditory learning in childhood to achieve the evolved pacific behavior of kinship that includes incest inhibition. Humans do not partake in incest if they are properly introduced to a nutritive bonding in the childhood period in which kinship with parents and siblings occurs as part of the human recapitulative process of mammalian evolution.

Incest is regressive human behavior of the most profound degree when the learning process of kinship, automatic to most other mammals, is deeply aberrant. Current investigations of incest disavow the Freudian theory that at one time in human history, incest was a norm. Psychiatrists point out that in nature, incest is very rare in animal behavior, therefore extrapolating that it never occurred in humans. In the dim past of hunting and gathering units of human existence with wide ranges of territory and great distances between other family groups, one is hard pressed to explain its absence. The very definition of *species* as "a naturally existing population of similar organisms usually interbreeding only among themselves" would attest to incest. Eventually, sexually active, genetically related young adults broke away from the dominant male with some of the incest reproduced female booty. They then formed clans of their own that eventually started to barter women in a process of maintaining clan identity without incest being obvious.

Nonetheless, modern explanations of kinship and the lack of incest behavior in the young suggest that the prohibition is innate and does

125

not require learning. While there is the genetic brain propensity for familiarity to develop into avoidance of incest, it doesn't take into account the learning that is necessary to reinforce its prohibition in the human. Neither do these explanations take into account the long history of rivalry between dominant males and younger offspring for sexual partners within a family or kinship environment. Not only is there the mythology from which to gather this evidence, there is the historical record in which a father, without the blink of an eye or the intervention of a legal process, could imprison his sons with a letter of cachet.

Freudian theory concerning incest came out of an appreciation of primal circumstances in which sexual rivalry existed between male members of an isolated family in a vast territory. Freud's Oedipus complex has been defined most clearly by Erich Fromm as he delineates its presence in human sexuality when the learning of kinship is incomplete. In the normal individual, while there is no real physical incest between parents and children, there is an emotional affective connection that cannot be denied.

"According to the classic concept a little boy at the age of five or six chooses his mother as the first object of sexual (phallic) desire (phallic stage). Given the family situation this makes his father a hated rival. (Orthodox psychoanalysts have greatly overrated the little boy's hatred of the father.) Statements like: 'When father dies I will marry mother.' attributed to little boys and often quoted as proof of their death wishes, are not to be taken literally because at this age death is not yet fully experienced as a reality, but rather as an equivalent of 'being away'. Furthermore, although some rivalry with father exists, the main source of deep antagonism lies in the rebellion of the boy against patriarchal oppressive authority . . . . He becomes afraid of him, fearing, specifically, that father will castrate him, his little rival. This 'castration fear' makes the boy give up his sexual desires for mother. In normal development, the son is capable of shifting his interest to other women, particularly after he has reached full sexual genital development about the time of puberty. He overcomes his rivalry with his father by identifying with him particularly with his commands and prohibitions."

In man's history, puberty is one difficult time. The male child goes from the kitchen of mother and sisters into the "long house keeping" of his father and other male relatives as an active process of learning male identification. If this transition does not take place, the male child remains with a character that is woman-dependent. "He continues to be fearful of men especially older father figures. He remains a momma's boy, a mother-fixated man who is narcissistic and spoiled with a deep feeling that he is wonderful and more important to mother than even his father.

He has difficulty making sound attachments to women and uses them as sexual objects of transitory gratification. In his choice of women, he looks for and elicits maternal behavior with his own dependent behavior that more often than not, drives the new mother-wife-companion to disgust and contempt."

In abnormal parenting, when there is war between partners, children often pick up the behavior that is propagated, and continue it into their own marriages. Incest begets incest; hate of the female begets hate of the new wife and visa versa. Pathology of relationships is learned generation after generation.

The normal limbic developmental period must be fully exercised by the parents in order for it to be internalized by the child. When shortcuts are taken in this development, the child acquires a pathologic sense of bonding with others that can reveal itself in all phases of bonding behavior. The many forms of pathology range from criminal sociopathic deviation to matters of dysfunctional mating and psychopathic social problems. Examples are necrophilia, serial killing of women, rape, child molestation, prostitution, incest, gender rejection, satyriasis, nymphomania, divorce, marriage as a recreation of a child-parent relationship, impotence, frigidity, Madonna-prostitute syndrome, and the Oedipus-Electra complexes.

Abandonment, punishment, rejection, engulfment and inappropriate attempts of showing love and tenderness with adult sexuality are detrimental parenting behaviors. With a defective limbic emotional character, the matured offspring become defective adults. The time frame for learning is most critical for kinship and bonding with family; the first three years are extremely important, but the process continues through puberty.

A child continues to absorb what a healthy or abnormal pair-bond *is* by parental behavior. Afterwards, what the child absorbs in the learning period regarding love between partners and siblings becomes the basis for its own behavior with mates and companions. A father or mother who is unable to reveal the forms of love beyond explicit seductive behavior or total rejection end up with wounded offspring who use the excuse that all they want is someone to love them, when, in fact, they are unable to love themselves or others.

Perhaps more obvious than incest as a result of poor nurturing is the immense personal, social and political problem of homosexual self-identity. In Western society prior to the wave of acceptance of homosexuality, how a child acquired a heterosexual self-identity was and remains, for the most part, a function of parenting. The physical establishment of an active gender is hormonally driven as a brain function, but gender self-identity is a separate brain learning process.

With the exception of those morphologic conditions in which primary sexual characteristics are genetically confused in sexual expression (hermaphrodism), it is anticipated a female or male mindset will arrive on the scene with the appropriate equipment.

Incest, homosexuality, other cited sexual abnormalities and the Oedipal problems are all related as variable degrees of an incomplete limbic development of self-identity. Our primordial sexual behaviors arise from our reptilian ancestors and continue to be modified by limbic brain functions; the long tortuous process of modification continues to produce social and psychological ills. The beginning of sexual behavior, the basis from which our sexuality is derived can be identified as the reproductive survival behavior of early reptiles who united only in aggressive sexual encounters.

In the evolution of meiotic reproduction that involved two organisms, the body of the organism evolved first. Gender came second. We observe in lesser animals behavior that tells us so. There are those special fish that can change their sexual orientation when a male is needed or a female is needed for reproduction. The behavior of an alpha neutered female canine that returns to male copulatory activity on its master's leg when the occasion seems to demand it is another example. Anatomical evidence can be ascertained by the evolution of the human sexual organs themselves as they embryologically differentiate into separate male and female characteristics from a single origin. Similarly, humans start as organisms in childhood without sexual differentiation in their limbic brains even though a peek at the external genitalia reminds us they are predetermined as how the limbic development should take place to make mind and body unified in behavior for reproduction.

Even when the pituitary gland of the brain starts up its engine at puberty, there must be a neural limbic component to compliment overt sexual behavior with the opposite sex. It is a limbic process initiated by parents. How does a child learn from its parents to be a female or a male? The process in the beginning occurs when a child gets a glimpse at what appears to be different between mom and dad. The first thing that comes to a child's attention is the external genitalia of each. Not too sophisticated child visual exploration tells, it has one like the male of the house or the female of the house. With language development, gender is reinforced with word symbolic markers that the child is a very nice "girl" or a very fine "boy". Consequently, gender words from the parents appear and validate visible differences. The child essentially assimilates its mental gender from its own observations as well as the verbal suggestions of parental definition. These stimuli are further reinforced with the dress codes of gender and parental segregation that begin early on. Then the parent begins the promotion of behavior that has been culturally established as male typical or female typical. Boys don't get to play with dolls and girls are not encouraged to play with knives and toy soldiers even though there may be "natural" tendencies not to do so. Children learn very early that first mother and then father can provide physical not sexually explicit limbic behavior of touching and holding, kissing and hugging, absolute precursors for adult heterosexuality. Heterosexual self-identity doesn't go as planned for reproduction if the parents do not take a proper place in this learning process. Since some individuals arrive on the parental labor force with their own sexual orientation problems, they become defective parents. Take the case of a female child who became a lesbian due to her parents' inability to nurture her heterosexuality.

CASE HISTORY: B. O.

B's mother was thought by her parents to be inferior due to her gender. She was not given the privileges of her brothers; she was denied a presence in her family in many ways and grew to adulthood with a sense of envy and contempt for men in general. She easily aligned her feelings with the then beginning movement to give women the right to vote and to attain the same privileges as men in the social-economic structure of society. She was drawn to marry a farm lad from a large family in which he had little emotional interaction with his European parents. Shy and not comfortable with females, he was attracted to the strong maternal dominance of the woman he married, B's mother, who used sex to acquire a husband not to enjoy one.

When B was born, she was an immense disappointment to her mother because she was not the designated and expected first born male. Her birth evoked a persistent rejection of the child that could not be assuaged by her father who had few skills of his own to be warm and accepting of a female. There was no love from the mother and a defective love from the father. B could not easily identify with her hostile, rejecting mother and could not be treated by her father as a girl child to love in acceptable ways of holding, kissing and touching. She could not make the subconscious neural limbic resolution of her gender as being that of her mother's. In analytical terms, she could not "identify" with a female parent. Over and over again early on in life she found subconsciously that it was her gender, the vital part of emotional self-identity that was rejected. To gain love that could calm fears and anxieties of childhood and eventually adulthood, she acquired masculine behavior to get superficial acceptance from her mother and from her father.

B's mother related to her girl child in a distorted limbic recapitulation of the basic reptilian sense of sexuality, as a competitor for her territory and the control of her mate. Gaining a modicum of love only through taking on the role of a male child, B became an unusual athlete who acted like a boy. She carried on a painful lesbian life in which she was unable to maintain lasting relationships even with other women.

Of related interest to the many aberrations of sexual maturation is the understanding of how a child develops an Oedipal character. It is just a more socially accepted variant of abnormal heterosexual maturation. In analytical terms related to the Freudian theory of the Oedipus complex previously defined by Fromm, the male, for example, cannot "transfer" from his mother and go on to "identify" with his father. This is a process brought about because of the mother's own defective sense of sexual identity. She unconsciously sees the male child, especially the first born, as an (penile) extension of her thwarted female self-identity. The male child is excessively controlled one way or another by her; she won't release the male child to the control of the father who may prefer to reject the male child for his own Oedipal-reptilian reasons. The momma's boy, as Fromm has already reminded us, becomes a defective mate and parent unable to be a loving, enduring husband and father. The Oedipal male is not a hardwired homosexual, but an incomplete heterosexual, child-like in his views, bound to a mother-dependent mentality and unable to be secure in any mature relationship with others.

An earlier question presented to the reader in this chapter asked if sexual identity as part of the evolved limbic brain's function required normal parenting to achieve normal heterosexuality. I believe the question has been definitely answered in the affirmative. *Normal, in this regard is not a cybernetic cookie cutter expression of the term, but a fluid moving mass action of change in human character. Within this process of normalcy, there are a head, a tail and a body with many shapes. Therefore, in Western cultures, what is normal regarding heterosexuality at this point in evolution is in a great flux. But with regard to the great middle, normalcy now includes an individual's mental acceptance of physical gender with respect to being attracted to the opposite sex.*

With such an assumption, heterosexuality can be considered a limbic brain function of survival related to reproduction not only in the sex act in which reproduction is possible, but also in the caring and in the well-being of the reproductive result, the offspring. To continue a successful survival through reproduction, the species attempts to reproduce offspring with characteristic physical and mental attributes of species. This automatic short process in most other animals is a lengthy complicated process of parenting in humans. For our purposes this aspect of human self-identity for survival is based on a normal recapitulative maturation of a child provided primarily by parenting. It allows for behavior that is not just the raw character of reptiles and the modified interests of old mammals, but it includes the extended parenting process of modern humans to develop independent progeny.

An individual's character, personality and emotional self-identity are first acquired from others and internalized to be its own in a process of cleavage (introjection) from an external environment of humans, called parents. Parents play a vital role in teaching a child *what to be emotionally* in terms of both limbic and reptilian behavior. Therefore it is important to include the part of reptilian-limbic self-identity that is acquired as a member of a family.

The observable behavior that characterizes an individual's character and personality as normal or abnormal with respect to basic emotions of love and hate learned during early family life can be identified analytically by professionals and others who can recognize subconscious emotional behavior. But for each individual, the subconscious part of self-identity is seldom appreciated by the word symbolic thinking part of an individual's brain. It is such a vital part of the self for survival that no matter what shape it acquires during the learning period in which parents and siblings are involved; it is subconscious and becomes almost immutable thereafter.

The subconscious characteristics of the emotional element of self-identity can not be described by an individual in terms of what he thinks his character is unless he learns about it, usually from others. This classic conscious/subconscious duality of a human is easily appreciated by the personal want ads found in most newspapers. In attempting to present themselves as potential mates or partners, these individuals disclose in their ads only what they consciously think they are. For example: "SWF, highly intelligent, likes to have fun and enjoy life to the fullest." The dark side of the individual, the unconscious contrary element that provides the deep emotional character of the individual is not appreciated. "SWF" has no idea that she hates men that try to dominate her.

Reptilian/limbic characteristics of each human, the principal emotions of fear and anger, love and bonding, are learned by the human from his early childhood experiences usually within a family. While emotional imprinting is mostly non-verbal and associated with the right hemisphere, as children mature and experience their status within the family, they also learn an automatic script of the auditory cortex. How the parents define the child, how the child reacts to this definition of self within the family structure and finally what the parents think about the world are retained dialogs that are repeated into adulthood.

Curiosity about the limbic emotional self began long before Freud's interest in child-parent relationships in the evolution of philosophical thinking about the importance of becoming human. It continues and is interesting due to the work of post-Freudian investigation; especially the groundbreaking work of J.D. Laing who unraveled much of the etiology of schizophrenia as a problem of inappropriate family relationships. He observed that the parents of schizophrenics did not understand that their role was to rear children to independent maturity and was not just to create a perpetual member of the family structure as children had been viewed thousands of years ago. What Laing's interviewees failed to understand in their roles as parents were the objectives that they were to nurture offspring first to be members of the family hierarchy in order to survive, and then to be adequate long term partners and parents living independently from their original family.

An individual who is thrust into the real world of competition cannot be successful as a dependent child, a dependent mate or an immature parent. Defective limbic parenting does not result in schizophrenia alone, but also contributes to most of the maladies of marriage and to sociopathic and to psychopathic behavior. In the convoluted knot of brain neurons once thought to be a matrix of continuous, uninterrupted connections, emotional self-identity for survival can be better defined as distributed brain systems of neurons that must be stimulated and modulated in a healthy manner for each newborn. In reference to failures called schizophrenia and other mental difficulties with characteristics of pathological dualistic personality, the anomalies have to do with the abnormal parenting of a child that then acquires abnormal unconscious emotional behavior of its own. This is a defective neurological process of union between the right and left hemispheres of the brain. The abnormal unconscious emotional visual self of the right hemisphere has a defective relationship with a defective left auditory hemisphere in which abnormal behavior is deceitfully denied or actually not appreciated at all. The developmental role of the limbic system must again be stressed as the prime modifier of our reptilian brain system that houses our basic *kill or be killed core of reproductive self.*

Freudian theory regarding the Oedipus complex must be given a renewed credit. We can now identify that Freud's clinical observations of parent and child behaviors provide a vital step in the understanding of the evolving function of the limbic brain in humans. The mammalian brain in humans continues to inhibit, however imperfectly, the primordial reptilian instincts of both children and parents to see each other as rivals in an ancient, once appropriate, drama of evolution.

Chapter 4

THE SIMIAN ELEMENT OF HUMAN ONTOGENY

HOW THE RIGHT CEREBRAL CORTEX OF THE BRAIN DEVELOPS.

MONKEY BUSINESS

The young men had different faces. Their torsos had their own individuality as well, but in spite of those differences, they had a defining similarity as they stood in cowboy postures without the chaps and boots, but with the Levi's and the swagger and the tooth picks bobbing up and down. While a few were squatting, others were perched on marble hallway stairs; one had a leg tucked up held by his encircling arms. This was a privileged class of boys, all freshly shaven even though it was only necessary to get that way every other day. Some of these enviable males had facial acne under inadequate treatment and most sported haircuts for crewmen. They were all jocks at Lewis and Clark High School in Spokane, Washington in 1949. David Kaminski, with a letter sweater he never wore, was not at all certain he was one of them.

The corps identification of these teenage athletes was a letter sweater, in a way, a testament to Samurai warriors and Knights of the Round Table. Letter sweater uniforms were not mandatory for daily wear, but the temptation was there to provide an ongoing parade of class distinction.

These guardians of variously shaped athletic balls were in a visual synchrony accompanied by a hushed babble, "Look at those tits, what an ass, boy, would I like to get into her pants." The vets were in their rape, rob and plunder phase. The season for a particular kind of ball was over; they were the victors of a battle over territory that didn't change hands. Their enemy, the athletes across town, had been vanquished. It was a time for getting their rewards.

Mary Lou Palmer, the object of their interest, unbeknownst to them, was not going to let it happen. Her pants and what the boys in those days called "a cherry" would remain hers for an extended period of years even though she was forever being sought after. She had already been swept off her feet by her own reflection. A trip-tych set of mirrors in her own private bathroom allowed her vision to reach round to an elegant back, give side shots and full body shots of other assets. A concave hand mirror revealed a dearth of oleacious pores, just peach fuzz. Posing at just the right angle, she could watch the glimmering sheen of her auburn hair following the directions of the pig-hair brush's grooming. The admiration took endless hours that never felt like indulgence. There were mouth exercises with pursed lips ready to kiss, peek a boo hints of smiles, languid open mouth displays of perfect upper and lower teeth. She created endless displays of pout accented by variations of pink, red, metallic border tones, magenta and violet lipsticks. She would study nuances of eyebrow elevation and the twists of her neck and a million other seductive postures front and back. "Mary Lou, it's ten thirty, time to go to bed."

Mary Lou was the object of her own admiration in a public theater that otherwise could have provided a legitimate audience. She created her own photo shoots that required no staff. Her own eyes became the photographer's camera. The pictures taken required a reflecting surface of a glass door or window. It was hard to get eye-to-eye attention. No male was safe taking a look at her celestial self from behind. She was quick to dart a look of disapproval which caught the culprit stealing her own action. Mary Lou was indeed in love with herself, because the modern human species has evolved a self that recognizes its own reflection is not someone else. She was narcissistic but not Narcissus.[1] Mary Lou's self-absorbing behavior was not the case with early hominids possessing triune neo-mammalian brains that had acquired a greater visual memory of retained images.

---

[1] In the myth of Narcissus, a handsome young man fell in love with his own reflection in an enchanted pool. Mistaking his own image for a water spirit living in the fountain, he was unable to capture his elusive love object. As he attempted to kiss it or embrace it, the image would disappear in the rippled waters only to return to taunt him with an expression of sadness. *Bulfinch's Mythology: The Age of Fable*

Terms

Prosematic communication: Non-verbal vocal, body or chemical
    signaling
Mimesis: Imitation or mimicry
Isopraxis: Two or more individuals exhibiting physical actions of a similar
    nature in unison
Echolalia: Immediate repetition of words spoken by another
Echopraxia: Immediate repetition of body movements by another

Early hominids had evolved to have a visual intelligence that exceeded less evolved species of simians who were threatened by their own reflections. They were bound to hostile dramas with their own images that appeared to be rivals or enemies. More advanced, evolving hominids, when viewing their own images in reflective surfaces, began to see others like themselves, not enemies. They certainly did not see an individual self. There was no symbolic verbal brain intelligence that could talk light rays and reflections and virtual images. Nor was there yet a brain that later considered those reflections phantom spiritual manifestations similar to what a human shadow was long thought to be.

Certain species of contemporary monkeys are believed by some to have a sense of human individuality wherein a mirror provides an image of an individual monkey self, just as a human recognizes his own image in mirrors. In this evolutionary proposal, it is most unlikely that without human interaction these modern monkeys do not appreciate their images in mirrors as being a specific reflection of their individual self-identity. They really do not think like Mary Lou. They really don't see "a self". As members of a society of monkeys, they cannot appreciate the image in the mirror as a single self. These monkeys have not evolved to appreciate images of individual self-identity, but only of a gang or troupe sense of a visual self. These more visually advanced monkeys who don't see monkey enemies in reflections, see other friendly monkeys as they would see them in their real environment as part of a troupe-society. They are separate monkeys only with respect to the degree the simian animals have achieved self-identity. They have their individual body-self and a higher visual-intelligent sense of self than the old mammals before them. Their visual brain sense of self was a gang sense of self. They were comrades, friends other guy-girl monkeys to pal around with. The subordinate mature males worked the territory of their hierarchy like crows intimidating a brown hawk. They have a unit identity of a trained drum corps. Normal for monkeys is what humans do when they regress into a mob mentality.

135

Similarly in a visually dominated mentality with very limited auditory language, early hominids behaved more like monkeys than anything approaching human status. They also misinterpreted what they saw in a placid pool. After quenching their thirst from cupped hands, they saw not an individual self, but another human from the same clan, familiar and comfortable to be around. "But" you say, "the modern monkey pats the top of his head and examines his own teeth and protrudes his own tongue for self-examination." It can be argued that visually dominant early man, as well as contemporary monkeys of this sort, displayed the quintessence of monkey behavior, visual mimicry. He could do it so fast and so in tempo with other monkeys he didn't know which monkey, the real one or the reflection of one was initiating the motor behavior. It was an intricate example of monkey see, monkey do; a pas de deux of visual mimicry in which the real monkey had no idea that he was not following the exact actions of the virtual monkey. Early visually advanced primitive man wasn't a self either, he was a clan self, not an individual. In his body, he had individuality, but not in his head.

An interesting experiment has recently been conducted by psychology professor, Dr. Mark Howe, of Canada's Lakehead University. He has been studying first childhood memories for nearly two decades. His research concludes children are first able to identify visual mirror images of themselves at eighteen months. These children are also thought at that age to have the onset of image retentive memory of recent past events. This research points out initial visual-image retentive memory begins in children who have developed a "me" sense of self. The researcher concludes that the advanced ability to remember, what he calls "autobiographic memory" is achieved only after a sense of self or "me" memory begins. This conclusion appears to be flawed. Visual memory does not begin with the child's ability to understand auditory language but precedes it. It is only when the child understands auditory language that he can report his visual memory.

The children in this study had already begun the sensory development of auditory symbolic language and had accessed a rudimentary verbal sense of self because they could understand the commands of the experimenters. "Who has a mark on his nose and who has a funny nose?" was asked of the children when they looked at mirror images of themselves after a splotch of red paint was placed on their noses. Although this study required no verbal response but merely a simple body response from the children, the young subjects still had to understand the auditory commands of the researchers. As these children demonstrated, the visual sense of self very quickly develops a childhood memory, but this memory is not identified until auditory language is partially or fully developed to access it.

While there are definite observations of isopractic group behavior in lower animals such as the reptile, this behavior is more representative of primates. Less sophisticated isopractic behavior is also appreciated in less evolved animals such as fish and birds who possess isopractic behavior in unyielding rigid genetic memory after millions of years of evolution. But the kind of isopraxis one sees in Los Vegas show girls in their all together is easily learned in its echopractic form observed in children trying to visually learn new motor acts.

Mimetic behavior evolved in monkeys as a byproduct of their more evolved visual-motor brains. They began to use more precise body language. Facial muscles developed and gave a greater breadth of expression to body language. Out of this visual brain of primates, hominids advanced to have a right cerebral dominance over prior evolutionary brain functions of reptiles and old mammals. The dominance was also over the left auditory cerebral hemisphere that was simultaneously evolving with greater size to create the different cranial features that separate humans from primates. The hominids began to develop frontal lobes and to acquire foreheads, but their behavior continued to be controlled by the visual right hemisphere.

The modern child recapitulates this evolutionary event until he becomes left hemisphere dominant, when his body actions begin to be controlled by word symbols, not visual cues. Prior to auditory language achievement, the child is directed by visual stimuli that very early take the form of mimesis with acts of isopraxis and echopraxia and eventually echolalia in the learning of motor acts that produce word symbols. Until the child masters his auditory skills, he is a visual being, whose character is being determined by what he sees and assimilates into his own right visually dominated brain. It is this visually silent part of the human brain that becomes the invisible part of the self, the anima-animus, the dark side, the unconscious shadow of humans. Unless this huge evolved component of self becomes identified by the left auditory symbolic brain we call the mind, we are unaware of that part of ourselves.

The human child starts learning quickly with his visual intelligence committed at birth but not fully developed; the child deserves the rightful description of a copycat. When we use the term "model", we think of a standard of imitation or comparison. When we use the term in psychology as in "The parent models for the child or the child needs a role model.", we refer to the visual and auditory mimesis and isopraxis adults and older siblings evoke in very young children. The process goes on without any inducement to do so. The learning essentially is involuntary. Parents, siblings and cohorts are instructors for early behavior if they like it or not. Children from early on imitate their parents' behavior and if not fully developed in auditory language, they perform body language just like their models. They learn the expression and circumstances for emotional awareness and display. They learn the way to look and be in terms of a personality. "Your father used to hold his head that way . . . You act just the way your mother used to act.", say the mates who learn to observe their partners after having known their parents. Young, visually impressionable children learn what visible body—facial expression goes with what emotion. Mimicking their parents and elders, they automatically assimilate a system of responses to emotional events without knowing it happened. (See Laing for the subconscious development of character or personality acquired during early family life in *The Politics of the Family*.) Neither the children nor the parents are conscious of the process.

This element of human self-identity derived from simian ancestors continues on to find a hero to emulate. If adolescents are caught up in gangs, the gang leader takes that role. It is the nonverbal monkey in our mental origins that makes the peer group so important to the adolescent in role modeling. Professional athletes, movie stars, rock stars or rap artists are often adopted as the mascots or idols of these groups and are emulated in their manner of dress and in their behavior. Most humans go on to fall in love with just one other person and stop seeing themselves in terms of a group. But the first recognition of the love object is still a right visual brain function that sees a subconscious reflection of itself.

The epoch of Freudian investigation of the subconscious created a new language for illness. Pressured by the medical discipline of thinking in terms of diseases and pathology, to gain acceptance within the field of medicine, mental states were given new names of psychosis and neurosis as if they were diseases akin to the diseases of the body. The entire world responded to these new terms and "the ego" and its defense mechanisms became common vernacular and defined an era of Freudian thought.

If, however, we take an evolutionary view of neuroses, we can appreciate that neurotics are really not ill as we know it, but think in less advanced forms of civilized thought processes. They actually represent older ways of thinking that were common to civilizations of the past. The well-appreciated ego defense mechanism of neurotics called "projection" can be defined as a primitive, visually dominated way of thinking. In addition to seeing ourselves in others, we see behavior in others we don't like when, in fact, the behaviors are quite characteristic of our own way of behaving. Yet we can't see ourselves in the sense of being conscious of ourselves in the words of our minds. We see ourselves, usually disapprovingly only in others. We "project" our behavior especially when it is associated with emotional sentiment on others. It also remains a way of thinking not only when observing body behavior of others, but also when we accuse others of thinking certain things when we are the ones that are actually doing the thinking.

Projection of one's thoughts on others occurred in distant humans that had not yet developed a more intelligent way of thinking in words. Without the intelligence of word symbols it was a matter of mixing object and subject because of association. (We still appreciate that cause and effect are not always related to the proximity of two events.) Early humans mixed up object and subject because they had not evolved word symbols that could differentiate the object sense (you or it) from the subject self (I or me). That concept came only with the evolution of words that defined separateness. Early inner body sensations were conditioned to outer object sensations, especially smells, sights and sounds of objects that stimulated our basic emotional survival needs. This inability to separate object from subject got things terribly mixed up and what was going on inside was thought to be a part of what was appreciated externally. A separation of the inner emotional sensation and the object out there in the environment took a long time to evolve in the mind of man. The separation of object and subject came about only after visual and then auditory symbolic neurons evolved to define the events as separate. (Today, we study situations by defining dependent and independent variables of an experiment that would have perplexed our ancient forefathers. See illustration in chapter with cave man and wolf.)

Projection is an immature and a former way of thinking from which blame and fault arose. Those that continue to blame and fault others without seeing their own involvement in the interaction can never solve the newer problems of a much more complex society. The process of adversarial law will not come down easily. Blame and fault have a hierarchical tone that someone is right and someone is wrong. It provides for both parties to remain in their self-proclaimed, reptilian-driven states of dominance. No one yields; there is no compromise, no logical change. The parties remain egocentric and unyielding to change and consequently dependent upon less evolved and less independent mental ways of survival. Successful compromise should be the characteristic of all just laws, societies and relationships.

Our silent visual self-identity can be appreciated to have evolved from the ability to communicate in the body language of monkeys in which signals to others occurred by physical changes in posture and facial expressions as well as color signals i.e. gray backs and red rumps. The basis of these body signals has an ancient origin that preceded primates as evidenced by the posturing of octopuses, but body language became foremost and the primary means of interaction in primates. Eventually, from the visual cerebral self-identity of primates, early humans evolved visual hand signals, then sign language using the arms and hands. These visual symbols were later transcribed in petroglyphs and finally into written visual symbols called hieroglyphics that expressed more complex objects and acts.

In the history of writing, pictographs and hieroglyphics slowly have been taken over by a phonetic alphabet in western cultures. Modern oriental language continues to use a more complex visually derived process to express man's written intentions that originate in both visual and auditory cerebral hemispheres. While both western and oriental thinking have their own individuality in written expressions that utilize both cerebral hemispheres, the evolution of both has developed wherein the auditory symbolic brain has come to dominate the visual brain and all other brain functions. Today, the impact of the right cerebral visual dominance of human behavior of the past is revealed in the Japanese dramas of Noh and Kabuki.

Fourteenth century lyric Noh drama originates from Saruguku or literally "monkey music". These dramas are pantomimic shows wherein wooden masks are used to create the actor's character. The play is dependent upon visual symbolism. Kabuki are plays of a similar type for the masses in which vulgar subject matter is the theme. These plays are more easily understood, because the body language is more easily identified and less complicated than that found in Noh drama. Rather than obscuring facial visual signs of emotional content with masks and thereby relying on body movements to identify content, Kabuki plays use actors with bizarre make-up and the themes are more easily understood in terms of posturing and body movements. In either case, tableau is the climatic point of the drama in which a visually understood picture is represented by persons suitably costumed or posed. In the West, children are more entertained by pantomime than verbal plays as they also reflect the visual origins of our past way of thinking visually.

The evolution of the auditory symbolic brain dominance over all other brain parts in modern man has been so extensive that the silent, visual-ideational, the visual-motor (except for writing of word symbols), and the visual-psychical functions of man's behavior have become hidden. Man does not appreciate this vast part of his self-identity.

In the individual development of the visual silent self, the recapitulation of the evolutionary process comes to pass in variable degrees dependent upon how much a child is allowed to express himself in visual day-dreaming, fantasy and artistic creative expression. The self-identity that has the primary visual characteristics of the primate continues beyond reflections of mirrors and appears figuratively in the eyes of adults and through the eyes of early school classmates. Then this visual identity acquires a sense of belonging within a group that is identified by visual signs that include haircuts, tattoos, clothing, flags, and uniforms. Eventually a modern young woman comes to appreciate how her individual visible attributes fit into the cultural standard; a young man does the same in terms of what his own physical status suggests in society. This show of the self is only part of that individual. It does not provide total identification of that self which may be more or less than what is visible.

In advanced human evolution, the silent visual half of our sense of self possesses the potential of human creativity which in any new expression always challenges the dominance of the verbal mind that must decipher in words that creativity. Our audible side is not fully conscious of the "other" silent half. The silent half remains invisible in terms of word identification until neurons of word symbols unite with neurons of visual symbols of the self. This unification of the components of the self creates a higher self-identity that makes it possible to understand the insight of a sage who proclaimed that vision is the process of seeing what isn't there.

Chapter 5

THE HOMINID ONTOGENY OF THE HUMAN SENSE OF SELF

HOW THE SYMBOLIC DUALISTIC SENSE OF SELF DEVELOPS.

Thomas, the autistic child

When he was born, Thomas was the apple of his father's eye. Dr. David Kaminski knew because he was Thomas' grandfather. Grandfather Kaminski had gone through the process himself as other fathers of sons had done when they looked under the swaddling clothes and confirmed, "It's a boy". Thomas' dad, David Kaminski's youngest son, changed the diapers of his first male progeny. He was a modern male who enjoyed such things as taking charge of warming the bottle and assessing the content's temperature on his wrist. He saw the first smile of the infant that told of the initial development of a socially complex brain. At age two, there were the joys of father and son in which Thomas was tossed into the air and on his papa's back he was given rides performed by the animal walk of hands and knees. Then something dreadful happened, Thomas would no longer try to catch basketballs nor would he toss them aptly toward a miniature hoop on the side of the garage. Thomas went underground. His mind stopped developing. The neurologist that examined him said he was autistic. Thomas' body was developing and his mind started to as well, but it stopped as if it had not been given the needs of proper food and a good night's sleep. Thomas was similar to other autistic kids. He seemed to be in a dreamy visual world of his own. He could not access the world of auditory language. The most important element of the human mind was missing. He did all the peculiar things autistic children do including "stemming", screaming outbursts of emotional sounds, behaving like a frightened animal and being unable to interact socially with family members. He would not make eye contact. He bounced up and down on his bed for extended periods of isolation while others played with their dolls and conversed in the babble required to stuff toy bottles of milk into rubber mouths. Thomas did not become an idiot savant, but he developed unusual intelligence that allowed him to work a computer most of the day. Thomas appeared to be schizophrenic, seeing hallucinatory images. In fact, when autism was first identified, it was known as childhood schizophrenia. Thomas' reality, his absenteeism was accompanied by staring and inattention. Thomas had to be snapped back with repetitive interventions of holding his head and calling, "Look at me!". Thomas was language deficient. At age twelve, his language skills persisted as a two year old just learning to talk.

"Tell Daddy 'hello'. Say 'goodbye' to Granddaddy. Say 'please'. What is this? Say 'car'. Thomas want some ice cream?" his father would ask.

And Thomas would reply, "Thomas want some ice cream."

Folks down in the psychology department of the local college would euphemistically say Thomas lacked language skills. What an understatement! Thomas' mind could not even think in words. He had no verbal thoughts of his own, but he was a seer of a primitive world of visual awareness and imagery. His mind had stopped developing at a time that recalls the evolutionary history of early man. Thomas, like his forebears, had acquired a visual memory of retained images, but no spoken language.

Verbal language begins around eighteen months in the child of a modern culture. At this time, other brain components of self-identity previously begun, continue to develop as well. The child has a beginning immune system of its own, a brain that appreciates pain, inside and on the surface of its body, an awareness of fear of body pain coming from taste, sounds, smells and sights. There is also an awareness of pleasant body surface and inner sensations with tastes, sounds, smells, and sights that inhibit fear of pain from those sensory sources. Then, too, an awareness of two specific facial images and voice sounds that inhibit pain and the fear of pain to the body from all sources come into being. More concisely, the child has started developing its immune system, its body sense of self, its reptilian sense of self, its limbic sense of self and its neo-mammalian sense of self. These brain systems of self have been entrained by two parents who are now responsible to stimulate further the development of auditory language. The new symbolic use of sound in the act of communication creates not only our highest intelligence but also a human double identity.

A double self became a human behavioral reality that is still not appreciated as a normal process of brain evolution. The process began when the symbolic auditory cortex evolved in the brains of early man. It specifically began with the evolution of the symbol that represented the human body. While the development of a brain that could utilize auditory symbols facilitated communication, it caused some bizarre side-effects of behavior. It created two neurological entities in the brain, one was the neo-cortex for the symbolic communication about the body, and the other was the neo-cortex that could define the body with respect to all of our other senses, especially the sense of vision. For reasons we have elaborated upon in previous chapters, it became an imperative of continuing survival to unite the two neurological neo-cortical components. What the body did had to be united to what the body was said to have done. The evolution is still in process wherein the neurological connecting is still going on as cultures strive to make humans responsible for their deeds. Unfortunately the joining process is not a wave crest of change, but one of chaotic assimilation occurring over hundreds of generations.

Likewise, a child's recapitulation of human phylogeny, is not simply linear development in which one new system gets completed before a second system has begun. Rather as new systems appear they must grow up together like siblings in a family. The analogy goes further; the systems have an effect on each other as they grow up as well. The child, therefore, has its own early limbic, reptilian and monkey self-awareness developing and maturing all interwoven complementing or inhibiting each other. In the development of auditory language, a child will take on what we will call *mind* self-awareness. It is the beginning of a second self-identity that exists for each individual in addition to what he finds real in vision and the other senses that deal with sensory reality of the body.* *Mind* awareness from the right auditory brain component that can speak, listen and think in symbols, without reinforcement by our other senses can be unreal, unsubstantiated. In the initial acquisition of words by the brain, they become real to us when our other senses confirm the meaning of the word symbol. The mind part of self-identity must develop beyond

---

* The evolution of visual symbols that stand for real objects in nature may have preceded auditory symbolic dualism. Early non-verbal man had his initial duality when he could draw a symbol that represented himself.

affirmation of words by other senses. To identify the symbolic self and the body self, the "I" symbol has come to represent all the sensations of the body as well as images in the brain. The auditory symbolic self, however, must become a prime mover of all previously developing senses of body self. It is a process that leaves some pathologically dualistic and other acceptably dualistic.

The adult says, "In my mind, I have an idea that will change things." The child at eighteen months has no such "I" that represents a separate body and a separate mind that is implied and understood by the adult speaker of the words. The child begins auditory language with a word that is not self, has nothing to do with self. "Ma ma" and "Da da" are words that are associated, neuron-connected, to the visual monkey part of its brain that identifies Ma ma's and Da da's faces in the right cerebral hemisphere. The twelve month old child begins to associate an auditory symbol with a face. Mother entrains in the infant's brain the first association of a monkey visual brain image with a human auditory brain sensory symbol. Watson and Pavlov would say it is a simple example of conditioning.* The neo mammalian component in the right hemisphere of the child's brain that recognizes facial patterns starts to join with the Hominid part of its brain that is just learning auditory symbols in the left hemisphere. Next, the child gets a more difficult assignment and must join by neurological conditioning a new word that Mother says. She teaches the new word, "Ba be". At first Ba be and Ma ma and Da da are all the same. They are word symbols associated in the child's miniscule mind with the two visual faces of parents. First the mother's face and then the father's face and eventually the visualization of their bodies become conditioned to the word "Ba be". There is no sense of self for the child at this stage of development except for what has already been described as developing in other systems. The child has a body-self that doesn't know about parents or its new mind-self. It has a simple brain that feels good when it hears the words, Ma ma, Da da, or Ba be. In monkey style, the child quickly begins to mimic words and facial expressions of the parents. It smiles back and tries to say the word symbols. The child is a visual and auditory pawn of the parents. At this time in development, the parents must entrain or stimulate the sensory auditory cortex of the

---

* Conditioning occurs as a result of observable behavior of an animal in which a response to a stimulus of one sensory modality, e.g. smell, is also able to elicit the same response from a different sensory modality, e.g. sound. Conditioning is a neuronal process of synaptic association of one cortex (smell) with another cortex (sound). Dynamic actions of neurons in which new connections interact with others make conditioning possible.

child. This is accomplished when the word "Ma ma" is conditioned to her smiling face. Then the child's newly developed sensory neurons of speech stimulate and hook up with newly developing motor neurons of speech on the left side of the brain. The process of learning to speak is continued by the child visually mimicking the appearance of the mother's mouth. She slowly speaks the word "Ma ma" moving her mouth in an exaggerated way so she can be seen as much as heard. After the child learns to speak the word "Ma ma", the child only does so when it hears from the mother the word "Ma ma". The child is still a pawn of the parents by only speaking the word after it is first spoken by the parents. The child acts as early clan Homo members behaved with new language; they needed to hear someone else say it before they could. Very soon thereafter, the child starts smiling at the parent before the parent smiles. The child has developed an internal neuronal connection between a visual right hemisphere cortical signal, the smiling mother, and a monkey cortical brain motor action of smiling. The child no longer needs to see a smile from an external source; the child learns to smile by itself. This is a neo-mammalian characteristic that occurs at the same time early language development begins. In a short time, the same neuronal connection occurs with the sight of the mother and the child's ability to utter the word, "Ma ma". Again, no need for further external entraining of this stage of language, there has now developed in the child an internal brain connection between an object seen in its visual monkey brain and a word symbol in its auditory symbolic brain that joins up with its own auditory motor cortex. This process enables the child to speak the word without assistance. In still more time, the child can say the word "Ma ma" that will stand for, actually symbolize the entire sensory awareness of its mother's body. This word "Ma ma" comes to be conditioned to all the comforts and lack of pain that the child's body appreciates. The child senses no separation of itself from this visible and now verbally symbolized object. The child's body sense of self is certainly separate from the environment in that physical pain which stimulates the body directly defines body limits. The child has no comprehension, however, that what it recognizes in the sights and sounds of parents and the word symbols of those sights and sounds are separate from itself. It has no idea of a separate mind, or self as we know it in our adult thinking brain. We refer once again to Levy-Bruhl, the anthropologist and psychologist, who reminds us that what is going on in the child at this time recapitulates a stage of early man before language fully developed. He could not really distinguish sensations of prey or predators from himself. He could only associate them with the sensations coming from his body; the excitement in his solar plexus and chest, the salivation associated with hunger for that prey. Modern man knows that his autonomic nervous system alarm sensations and his hunger sensations are separate from the animal of his regard. He appreciates that the separate animal caused the sensations in his separate self. Baby, like early non-speaking hominids, does not.

With greater language development, the child learns that its body has a generic name "Ba be". If there were a quintuplet of babies in the crib, they all would respond to the word "Ma ma" and would all feel that Ma ma was speaking to them because they were all called Ba be. The word symbol "ba be" then must go on to be appreciated in the child's mind as a greater sense of self-identity. It is this word symbol of self that creates a mental dualistic brain appreciation of what the self is. It is dualistic in the sense that what the mind says in symbols about the self can be separate from what the body does.

Symbolic language goes beyond being conditioned to mother's voice and face. Language provides an association between the body of the child and the name, "Babe". Children developing a generic word for their bodies are not separate individual bodies but a group of baby-bodies. The generic name "baby" refers to any baby in our contemporary language usage. The child appreciates it that way as well. It is separate only in the sense it is a *member* of a group and yet indivisibly mixed up in the group. The auditory (word) symbolic sense of self is as much the baby it sees next to it, as the one it sees in the mirror when mother holds baby up to see itself. The child does not really see itself. It sees another baby just like itself. This is a pre-narcissistic visual monkey sense of group self. The child learns a word symbol that moves from an association of comfort with a mother's face to a baby's face.

Generic names like "baby" are similar to the pronoun "you". After we teach children a generic word, it soon is used with early command words for body actions. "Baby sleep, Baby eat" is the talk of a generic or multiple self-identity of our ancestors. Baby is not an individual "I" self yet. Until the child learns "baby" is a symbol for his body alone he still is mixed up with other babies he can see and also with the word "ma ma" that is conditioned to all of his body needs. As early language symbols are learned, the child has already begun the development of greater visual memory that characterized early man who appreciated visual images in memory after the visual stimulus had passed. Soon the child can remember a picture and sound of its mother when she is out of sight. Unless asleep, full of milk, warm, comfortable in every way with empty and dry diapers, the child is back into its reptilian self. "Ma ma" is cried out in tantrums of full emotional timbre to bring her back into sight and service when body pain begins its assault on comfort.

As the eighteen-twenty month old child continues to exercise its earlier self-identities and learns the word "Johnny", the new identifying word refers to only one body, not any body. Given names were considered very sacred by Old Stone Age and New Stone Age peoples when they took names such as Running Bull or Killer of Snakes. In those very distant days, only heads of clan hierarchies acquired given names because given names were sacred and reserved only for those in command; given names were for royalty. Others who were members of a hierarchy under its leader, required only a group name; they were not important enough for a given name. They got the clan name which has changed over thousands of years from a totem animal to one we easily recognize such as "McCoy".

The new given name provided to a newborn becomes attached to a child's body actions and it becomes an internal circuit of the child's auditory symbolic nervous system. The child starts talking about itself in third person; "Johnny wants some ice cream." Mother continues to entrain new words, but now the child speaks its own given name that represents the body and the acts of that body. "See Johnny run", "See Ann sit." are not in reference to a mind, they refer to a body doing those things. Mind is unknown to the child. The child is not yet separate from the body in self-identity. When the child learns to use the pronoun "I", it still has not acquired a separate mind from the body; it still refers to body-self and all that we know has come to pass in that body. Even when Johnny is asked to remember and think, he still has the Johnny-body symbol connection that is doing those mental tasks. Only when the word "mind" is learned does it come to pass that the given name and the "I" are attached to a symbolic second self of the mind. When the child learns that it has a mind and a body, it recapitulates the event in man's history when early man began to use spoken and drawn symbols that established the awareness there was a spirit separate from his body.

Before the "I" comes along with a separate body, but not a separate mind, Johnny learns to follow commands obligatorily from parents. "Run, Johnny." "Go play, Johnny. "Eat, Johnny." Johnny does it all because he still acts like a primitive language developing human who doesn't have a complete sensory motor circuit in his language left brain that gives him a greater language derived sense of self. Part of the language self, the sensory part, is still in the brain of his parents. After he learns the sensory part, he still is a primitive human under the control of those that can give commands; he first can only respond to words, language symbols, that stand for his body actions. He then learns the motor part and eventually learns to speak the words all by himself. Then Johnny goes out in the front yard and says what he has just learned. He repeats what Mother says. "Sit.", he says to a younger kid, or a less developed one. "Get out of here.", "Stop that.", he says only what was heard and said to him. With a new fervor, he is able to say those words when those who said those things to him are out of sight. He will soon say to his friends to gain even greater respect and power, "Ma Ma says you should not do that". As the psychologist Jaynes points out, the child takes a recapitulated step that primitive man took when he heard voices of gods that commanded him to do things. At this stage of ontogeny, the child is still a word-language robot. He repeats what was put in his head. He has a simple prehistoric kind of a word-symbol mind.

Eventually by the middle of his second year, the child gets into what Mahler calls the "rapprochement stage of the separation individuation process". He fights back to authority. He refuses to go to bed when it's time; he becomes "negativistic", refusing to do as he is told, and in fact, he does just the opposite. "No" is stolen away from the parents' vocabulary; it is internalized in the child's own brain circuitry. He has a new power that is as profound as the stealing of fire from the gods. It is the same power that shook up the gods and the earthly leaders of hierarchies in ancient times. Learning to say "no" is either a tragic or heroic change in human language (mind) self-identity development. If parents don't allow children to exercise this new self-development of language, they condemn them to a personality that never can give up being a "dependent non-entity". Many parents see this new language of "No" as the emergence of a wild animal that needs more beating down to break its spirit. They see punishment as part of the civilizing process which if not undertaken, will be the beginning of a criminal offspring. Society still labors with this ancient idea that punishment early on is the only way to get a conforming member of its particular order. A child that is prevented from saying "no" develops into an adult who remains the ward of everyone that tells him what to do. He is selfless in terms we now can really understand. He has no self will, no sense of self in the language sense of self. He remains, as does his body, at the beck and call of spoken and remembered words of others. He becomes a robot of others doing their bidding without question or examination. It doesn't take much to sell him a worthless second-hand car.

On the other hand, the child that learns to say "no", stops that process and begins his own independence. The self, if given this chance, must continue to learn new horizons of language self-identity or get stuck in a limited way of handling life by saying "no" to any suggestion. He gets stuck in a limited way of thinking by always saying "No". This can lead to omnipotent contrary dependence on others because these people are just waiting for someone to suggest something so that they can say "no".

"What do you think about this Renoir?"

"I don't know. What do you think?"

"Well, I just love its style and its colors and its modern expression of objects."

"Well," says Miss No, "I don't. I just hate it. I hate Renoir." This limited language development in children who are not led past saying "no" results in individuals who are stubborn and blockheaded.

We now can see three types of humans that have been cast-typed from poorly developed auditory symbolic training in the sense of self. The first is a person who always does what he is told, a person who is highly suggestible. The second is one who repeats what others, especially authority figures, tell him to say. The third is a person that always says "no" and often does just the opposite of what others say, no matter what they say. These three types are at least better off and stand apart from those that did not receive even a fraction of this early language training. Individuals that don't get early language training that prepares them for the appropriate verbal conventions of society develop into real outcasts. They become reptile or old mammal equivalents, living in a world of wordless fear and profane anger.

More language development allows the child to recapitulate how his ancestors began to understand time, past and future. In this process, the developing language symbolic mind-self learns to lie about past and future actions. A perilous journey has begun for the child who is torn between a lie and the truth which is epitomized by the apocryphal statement of guilt by George Washington when he chopped down the cherry tree and could not tell a lie. A century later, another great man, Sir Richard Francis Burton, explorer, adventurer and translator of many languages, more accurately describes a young child's natural propensity for lying when he called himself a "resolute and unblushing" child liar.

The young child accessing auditory language loves to listen to stories, *ones you make up* or ones that are read from children's books. The new words children have learned stimulate big movies up in their little visual monkey minds. Those stories are as vivid as real events in the real world. Children at this stage are just beginning to appreciate reality, but are very much attracted to the world of make believe as were their Old Stone Age ancestors.

For Old Stone Age clan members, there was no difference between fantasy and reality. A story needed no proof especially after the more intelligent priests could tell by looking through a tiny stone aperture at Stonehenge that the sun would appear at a certain time to start planting. Predicting astrological events told the common folk that the living god-priests were actually controlling the transit of stars and planets. ("Golly, those priests know everything! No matter what they say, it must be true.") Old Stone Age clan members prior to their learning a new verbal concept of time, future and past, sat listening to their priest leaders like children not knowing the difference between reality and fantasy. However, the smarter priests knew the difference and held the lowly of the clan in check. The knowledge of time, past and future, was sacred stuff.

When the child starts using this important milestone in the auditory symbolic mind's development, he recapitulates the actions of those ancient priests. He starts saying things and it does not matter if there is any veracity. Everything he says is true. Then mom and dad come on the scene for a child's lesson in reality versus fantasy. Time gets started in his mind without the need for a wristwatch.

"Where were you when I called you to come in for your lunch?"

Buster, still in his pre-reality verbal mind says, "I was right here all the time. You just didn't see me."

After a few similar expressions of the child's new unbridled freedom of speech without verification, he learns a new word that is reinforced with a spanking or two. "You're lying. Go to your room until I tell you to come out." In the future, remarks to the child such as, "Where were you?" "Where have you been?" and "Get up to bed in a few minutes." are appreciated in their timely sense of reality. Without such training by a parent, a child will develop into an adult with a mind-body identity split irrevocably into a pathological two. Without the auditory language training to bind body acts to mind symbolic thought, a child never learns to stop what we once called his fantasying, but now we call his lying. The child will become an adult without a conscience. He will be called a sociopath because he lies about most of his actions. He has no emotional sense of regret or guilt that comes with the language development of learning not to lie.

A human who develops a symbolic auditory language sense of self in childhood, in a process of social development, is taught to be "a man of his word". This process is incomplete, and still ongoing. Many remain dualistically dysfunctional. The symbolic word speaking half of the brain is not completely or maturely connected with that other half of the brain that expresses visually and emotionally induced action.

After all, our ancestors took thousands of years to get the process activated. There was an epoch of normality in which early humans were dualistic and, consequently, very confusing and confused. The entire legal systems of Homo followed because humans were in a slow evolution of joining their symbolic auditory selves to their body selves. Proof of lying was a real problem for tribal chiefs who had no forensic knowledge and only witnesses who said what they were told to say. Rutherfurd tells of early tribes of England who in the determination of fault came to be judged always with one or more witnesses for both plaintiff and accused. The landed rank of a witness created truth based on his communal importance. Members of lower ranks, the peasants without land, were plentiful witnesses for either side of a problem. They would testify without truth the way they were instructed. The African Castor bean, also known as the truth bean to primitives, was handed out by chiefs to litigants. The rival who survived its lethal poisonous effects obviously was not telling a lie. It was real evidence that the truth of past acts was very elusive and lying was difficult to prove. As late as the 1840's in India, Burton described the primitive mind, while simultaneously identifying the duplicity of obsequious behavior that was but a guise for subversive thoughts and out right lies.

". . . a portly, pulpy Hindoo, the very type of his unamiable race, with a catlike gait, a bow of exquisite finish, a habit of sweetly smiling under every emotion, whether they produce a bribe or a kick; a softly murmuring voice, with a tendency to sinking; and a glance which seldom matched yours, and when it does, seems not to enjoy the meeting. How timidly he appears at the door! How deferential he slides in, salaams, looks deprecating, and at last is induced to sit down! Might he not be considered a novel kind of automaton, into which you transfer your mind and thoughts—a curious piece of human mechanism in the shape of a creature endowed with all things but a self."

Humans who successfully accomplish the task of uniting the symbolic mind with body actions do not develop the deceptive and dissembling behavior of the Hindu described by Burton. The normal socializing process, however, does allow us to remain relatively dualistic. We learn that "white lies" have a great deal of social value in a world that deals with others easily threatened by the truth about themselves or even the untrue opinions of others. We are able to remain that way because we have learned to talk to ourselves internally, silently without others hearing our inner thoughts. Children are chastised for expressing not only fanciful things, but also real things they observe. Out of the mouths of children . . . They are taught not to say out loud things that are asocial. All humans, to an extent, go underground at this time of developing language as a process of becoming socially adaptive. We continue to be normally dualistic without punishment in our present state of evolution not with respect to body actions but with respect to mind actions of speech. "Good morning, Mr. Nagele, my, you look nice in that tie." But under the breath of audible language, Ms. Sexually Harassed Secretary speaks her silent mind, "You dirty, old man, you."

From this ancient process of language development in the brain that creates a dualistic self-identity, Jung came to see all humans had dark sides to their character. A great number of his patients had hidden lives, asocial, evil and self-destructive. The varying hues of darkness developed in a poorly nurtured childhood in which the animal self was harmfully regulated and controlled by the word symbolic mind of parents and teachers. There was an incomplete neuronal binding of auditory symbolic and asocial body behavior.

In some individuals, this dark side is so threatening, so out of touch with the socially acceptable side of behavior, it remains inaccessible to consciousness. Most of this part of self-identity is a function of the right visual hemisphere connecting the emotional elements of self. Normal mind consciousness is aware of inner thoughts and spoken thoughts, but not necessarily of its early development of joining body, (the visual hemisphere) to mind, (the auditory symbolic hemisphere).

Colin Wilson draws our attention to the human's two basic selves. He gives us a glimpse of duality based on the work of Roger Sperry and Michael Gazzaniga who studied patients in which the corpus callosum or cerebral commissures are severed to control certain types of epilepsy. The corpus callosum is the structure that connects the two large cerebral hemispheres of the brain. These patients have come to be known as "split brained" because there is no connection between the speech and thinking brain of the left cerebral hemisphere and the visual appreciating brain of the right hemisphere. In studies of these patients who are allowed to view a naked woman, the visual side that emotionally appreciates the sight with giggles, is unable to tell an examiner why he is laughing. There is a block between the seeing and the talking parts of the brain. The block caused by the surgical disruption of the connections between the two hemispheres dramatically reveals the lack of neuronal connection between the older reptilian-limbic-neomammalian self-identity brain of vision and the human brain of auditory symbolic language. The neuronal connecting structure, the corpus callosum, while in place between both hemispheres, must develop new neuronal connections in early human development. These connections are not there automatically at birth but must be taught to children. The teachers entrain control of the behavior of the visual brain by the language side of the brain. The visual hemisphere, the monkey component of human self-identity, develops rapidly and is already connected to the limbic and r-complex (emotional) older brain components of self-identity when language begins in a child. Wilson states, "The right brain could be regarded as the gateway to the unconscious mind." He comments: "highly disturbed adolescents function like split brain patients, in the sense that the two halves go their separate ways." The psychopath and the severely autistic child are pathologically related. The autistic child has extremely poor language self-identity development; his primary sense of self remains in a rudimentary visual, neo-mammalian, early hominid hemisphere where he is motivated by phantoms produced by his visual memory. The psychopath is also mostly monkey, but with more of a rudimentary language self-identity in which he can talk and think in limbic and reptilian logic. He is pathologically dualistic and lies or hides in deceit as the connections between his monkey self and his language self are also incomplete. His language self-identity does not develop sufficiently to inhibit the antisocial elements of the monkey and older reptilian and limbic parts of his self-identity. When he is out of sight, he is his animal self. Within sight, he is a phony, compliant member of society who lies about his actions out of sight. The cerebral commissures and corpus callosum are a two way street in which actions from the right are connected to the left by means of neurons representing symbols for those actions that are visually and emotionally derived. It is along this brain intersection that the word symbolic mind blocks its animal behavior.

In addition to the observations of surgically induced split brained humans, the importance of binding by actual neuron synapses, the left auditory symbolic cortex to the right visual emotional cortex can be appreciated in the Phineas Gage Syndrome and victims of anosognosic strokes. The former, in which there is damage to the frontal lobes, results in personality or mind defects similar to a disconnection between right and left hemispheres. In this injury there are: 1) defects in decision-making and reasoning power, something we call "higher cognitive skills"; 2) lack of social appropriateness, (the ability to read others by appreciating that certain obtuse things said can hurt the feelings of others); 3) no inhibitions of egocentric behavior characterized by braggadocio, uncaring and cruelty toward others, being boastful and making remarks at the expense of others we know as "put downs"; 4) lack of feelings of empathy for others and the understanding of how others might feel if opposed to one's own convictions; 5) no understanding of another's position or being able to tolerate that position and negotiate differences; 6) a lack of a full range of affect in which the emotions are "flat" or "shallow" except for violent outbursts; 6) the inability to be independent and productive. Patients suffering from this syndrome do not experience a disorientation with time and place, nor do they suffer from any defect of intelligence regarding recall of facts. However, children who incur this kind of injury are especially defective in social development and eventually demonstrate a deterioration of social behavior.

Anosognosic stroke victims are similarly defective. These patients have right sided cerebral strokes that injure the left side of the body and result in a strange loss of understanding that the stroke side of their body even exists. They, too, acquire a flat affect, a lack of emotional regard of the loss, an inability to plan for the future, to make decisions or to foresee what is going to happen. They are unable to appreciate what has happened to them or what others think of them. Like the Gage syndrome victims, these patients also lack executive cognitive ability.*

What we see in common for these conditions is a dissociation of the mind (the cortex on the left that talks and thinks) with the body (the cortex on the right that gives consciousness regarding the body). In addition, there is a common defect of thinking and a lack of emotional expression to the talking left auditory cortex. The differences exist due to the degree of injury to the right and left sided union of the cortices. In the Gage syndrome, the union is disrupted only in the prefrontal cortex while in the anosognosic stroke victim, the entire hemisphere is essentially disrupted.

In normal subjects, the prefrontal cortex in the frontal lobes unites the right and left hemispheres for the purpose of executive cognitive functions. The ongoing evolution of human intelligence in this respect, depends upon both vision and sound that come together in the prefrontal cortices for the purpose of higher intelligence for survival; the ability to appreciate how others feel and to be able to negotiate with others without anger and resentment. All of the pathologic states mentioned previously demonstrate clearly to us that unless there is a joining of auditory and visual mental behavior, we remain at a disadvantage for the most evolved form of survival in which compassion, sharing and empathy play a role.

---

* Other examples exist of disconnections between right and left hemispheres. One involves a defective emotional quality to the spoken word as a result of right hemisphere brain damage. *Expressive aprosodia* is the clinical term that describes the condition in which the individual is unable to express common emotions such as joy, anger and sadness. These individuals speak in a flat, unemotional voice that often results in miscommunicated emotional messages. ("Effects of Two Treatments for Aprosodia Secondary to Acquired Brain Injury" *The Journal of Rehabilitation Research and Development* Vol. 43, number 2, pages 379-390, May/June 2006. The second example of a defective binding of the right and left hemispheres, akin to the insight of R. L. Stevenson in his *Dr. Jekyll and Mr. Hyde*, is a noninjurious instance of developmental-pathological duality described by Ben Macintyre in Timesonline (WWW. Timesonline.co.uk, December, 2006). His discussion of the personalities of double agents and moles clearly demonstrates that certain individuals have no problem living in two different worlds because of their split psychological make-up.

However, most analytical and contemporary Freudian psychological treatment of disturbed individuals tries to get them to understand the preverbal-emerging-verbal animal-unconscious traumatic history of themselves. The treatment attempts to change behavior by the process of insight. Too many therapies don't address the full neurological depths of the unconscious self, nor do they recognize that insights and recollections of traumatic mental events can't easily change the hard-wired mal-development of the dualistic mind. The therapies, while trying to drum up old memories of "trauma" and attempting to rehash or renovate old developmental processes, have met with limited success. Most therapies should be developmentally directed during childhood, not after the concrete has set.

From an anatomical prospective, Colin Wilson expresses an understanding of the conscious (verbal) and the unconscious (non-verbal) self with respect to cerebral hemispheres. Yet he concludes: "most of the theories of earlier psychologists-Freud, Jung, Adler et. al. are redundant." Nevertheless, early analytical psychology is from whence we came on our journey of trying to understand who we are. Now in disrepute, these analytical concepts still provide valuable steps in understanding how a mind develops. Revised thinking should not exclude the brave steps taken by others from the past. After all, Freud began the first serious awareness of our sub-conscious, actually our other self.

The left-brain hemisphere that creates sound symbols for communication results in humans that are initially dualistic, split, as if two humans. There is the individual self that is symbolized in language and the non-verbal-to-be seen body-self. Obviously, these two entities do not always act in a synchronous manner. This duality for most of us is one in which the language self is in control of the non-language, visual self. This control is completely disconnected in the split-brained individuals who have undergone surgery. In other humans, there is partial control we view as an abnormal schizoid mind. Those that are seriously abnormal are classified as schizophrenics or psychopaths. These individuals demonstrate a rudimentary lying type of control of the language left hemisphere over a disturbed right hemisphere in which both reptilian and limbic distortions exist as described in chapter 2 of this section. Then, on the other hand, there are degrees of neuronal disconnection and a lack of control of the language-thinking mind to a normal degree of sorts. These "normal" individuals appear synchronously united in body and mind, but they are only partially so depending upon the extent verbal mind development remains in control of the non-verbal, visual hemisphere. Symbolic-self development can remain partially connected with the visual, non-verbal self in degrees of normalcy. This non-pathological form of duality is characteristic of most normal individuals. When caught red-handed, there is an admission of guilt, a need for forgiveness. The deeply pathological form of duality, on the other hand, provides us with a person, not always a model citizen, but often an acceptable citizen during the day, and one who murders after dark. The dualistic process derived from language, develops in early childhood then becomes a way of life that is compatible with survival in society or one that results in severe asocial behavior that is not compatible. Modern societal members who consider themselves normal will most often tell the truth, but if things are just right, if they are certain they will not be caught, they will allow the body to do things the verbal mind would otherwise not allow. For the most part, we are in our "right mind", in our left hemisphere in control of the visual-motor-emotional connections in the other hemisphere, while psychopaths are never there. (For other extensive elaborations regarding the conflicts of right and left hemispheres read: *Poltergeist* by Colin Wilson, Nel Books, London: 1981.)

The duality occurs in adults as a result of how well or how poorly the reptilian, limbic, and visually dominant simian elements of self-identity are modulated in childhood. Some children being taught to control their reptilian-limbic-monkey selves are abused by parents and other authorities who use excessive corporal and verbal punishment. These abused children begin as retarded reptilian individuals who learn to live in the mental caves of total fear of the world. The abuse continues when they are caught in minor misbehaviors; they are punished now for not just body acts but for symbolic denial we call lying. The retarded entrainers have no good ideas regarding the successful way to bring about joining verbal-language (mind) and non-verbal, visual (body). By being too heavy-handed with punishment, these parents never reward children for telling the truth about their asocial body activities. These children cannot win; they are always punished if they are found out not telling the truth or are punished after telling the truth. Sir Richard Burton, a self-admitted childhood liar, stated: "I could never understand what moral turpitude there could be in a lie; unless it was told for fear of the consequences of telling the truth."

Children's fears of the consequences for doing right or for doing wrong lead to extremely frightened adults who develop loner type personalities, inferiority complexes as well as those that have schizoid personalities, multiple personalities and psychosis. If, on the other hand, there is not an appropriate suppression by entrainers of the emerging reptilian self-identity and there is not guidance at the appropriate time in a child's development in which corporal punishment is needed, children emerge as reptiles acting out their fears in ruthless anger. Two distinct abnormal dualistic types of humans emerge from this process: those that spend their lives seeking approval by being fearful of others and those who don't give a damn and kill without any regard for approval. In either instance these individuals remain with a talking external side that covers the tracks of the hidden side.

R.D. Laing, in *The Divided Self*, first described this dual self-identity from his observations of psychotic patients. They actually experienced themselves as primarily split into a mind and a body when they were going crazy or were just beginning to be crazy. They experienced themselves prior to extreme deterioration as being their "bodies" and not being their "minds" because they sensed the mind was being lost. Actually they were selves originating from the body right hemisphere observing a progressive deterioration of mind in the left hemisphere. The split that the patients felt, Laing was able to observe in their language behavior which demonstrated an actual physical neurological disconnection of one part of the brain from the other. It was a breakdown of the neuronal union of the left hemisphere with the right. These very sick individuals found themselves at the mercy of a prehistoric rudimentary thinking mind afraid of everything and angry at every human thing. Their primary self-identity was not in the left auditory hemisphere but in the right visual monkey-child hemisphere. Their language was not rational and not linear but stunted and poorly connected to the visual-body brain hemisphere. When the stunted individual with a poorly connected union was subjected to too much stress in life, the neurological union actually underwent a regressive disassociation. Stress for these individuals was too much undischarged fear that the mind-body union broke down.

Many modern humans appear to be fully connected. They appear to be just what they say they are and do. Laing, however, describes many humans who are not really what they appear to be but are not necessarily schizophrenic. They really do not have their total selves controlled by the in-charge, executive decision-making, self-identity of the left language hemisphere. In reality, they are faking the process, pretending to be in their "right minds", left hemisphere controlling the acts of body and mind. These individuals that comprise the majority of adults in the modern world have an abnormal "passing" form of duality in which they are perceived as whole. They actually operate out of the right monkey-child-body side. Laing describes this form of a divided personality as a self with a false-self trying to pass as normal. Their excessive needs to be dependent drive them to be complaint. As children, they never have had the opportunity to be real because they have been left alone, actually abandoned or excessively punished. These children have never been rewarded for telling the truth about their asocial body activities. They can not win; they have always been punished if they lie or tell the truth. Individuals not reaching a full left brained control of their actions continue to provide society with a persistence of an evolutionary brain process that can only be hurried along by understanding its true need for nurture.

Chapter 6

VERTICAL INTEGRATION OF HUMAN SELF-IDENTITY

HOW THE EMOTIONAL AND HIGHER INTELLECTS ARE
INTERRELATED.

Multiple selves

Mrs. Dedra Moore was in Dr. Kaminski's examination chair. Her right leg was crossed over her left; the right was oscillating in a staccato of movement suggesting a mind state of perturbation. Dr. Kaminski was behind in his schedule. He was being true to the tardy reputation of the medical profession. Kaminski's glasses were pushed up against his nose a bit further than usual to feign composure. Looking cross-eyed just for a moment at his patient's chart, he commented, "I see you are Nadine Angstrom's mother. Nice to meet you." The doctor and his patient began their first encounter.

The patient's animosity that Dr. Kaminski recognized in her legs but not her words would soon be forgotten. It was not just something he hoped for; he was confident a successful transference would make this new patient an old one who would return again. The biased process in Kaminski's favor would not be accomplished because of his unique skills of handling patients, but because the process had an ancient history in which patients obligatorily gave themselves over to their priest-physicians. Patients were not independent minds when they surrendered to their healers. They were reduced to subjects following imperative commands.

They were in the shaman's spell. Kaminski was going to observe how Mrs. Moore managed this transformation of self as he plied his trade. Mrs. Moore's angry beast inside her began a metamorphosis into a dutiful child who took Dr. Kaminski's commands without resistance. Her voice changed into sweet tongue-tied utterances. She also squirmed and began a body movement of acquiring more comfort on the now warm seat of the examining chair. Up just a bit on one side of her pelvis and then on to the other, it appeared to be a sexy wiggle. Then the right leg lost its position of dominance and the left demurely came forth to rest on top of the other. Unlike women who crossed their legs and primly adjusted their skirts downward, Mrs. Moore tucked up her skirt to reveal, not conceal her thighs. Kaminski's and his patient's eyes were deadlocked during the process. Both pairs were watching to see any change in the fusion of sight. Kaminski held on for dear life. Those legs were fine weapons of social combat. He knew better than to lose his position of control with a reflexive male peek at leg anatomy. When the examination was finished, the seductive child quickly vanished. In a platoon sergeant's voice Mrs. Moore started asking questions about what transpired. It was time for the cross-examination in which she took charge and began questioning the doctor. "What did you mean when you said the arteries were normal? Uh huh, do you think I have high blood pressure?" Kaminski held on again. Here, before him, was a different Mrs. Moore, now mature and stern. "What was going on inside," he eventually asked himself. "What pressure was coming from Mrs. Moore to make you feel so uncomfortable? What made you feel the need to hold on? Hold onto what?" Kaminski wasn't playing doctor for Mrs. Moore, he reasoned, he was simply being a doctor for her. He finally appreciated that his presence was a threat to Mrs. Moore's well being and she was trying to manage the stress of being under his control. He appreciated that her management was stressful to him as well. After all, Mrs. Moore was a very attractive woman.

The vertical organization of self-identity is established in the nervous system by *distributed systems* of neurons that mediate a specific behavior. They are also called neural networks, assemblies or pools. There is an ascending layered architecture of increasing complexity of these systems in the brain deceptively including lobes and hemispheres in which incoming sensory neuronal impulses cause excitatory or inhibitory synaptic potentials.

Humans don't have the through and through natures of good guys or bad guys portrayed by some novelists; they are capable of a full menu of possible personality behaviors typical of less evolved vertebrate animal types including humans of the distant past. The lower local circuits of neurons within each distributed personality system of the self that represent less complicated vertebrate animal types and humans can be stimulated to produce their characteristic behavior or bypassed to reach higher distributed systems of more sophisticated self-identity. Between each level of a given distributed system of self-identity, there is the capability for a graduated or modulated expression of characteristic behaviors. This modulation is brought about because the synaptic interaction of neurons provides for integration between each level of self in a combined function of reciprocal inhibition of one system and stimulation of another. One appreciates the harmony of this modulation in the gradual process of becoming slowly irritated at someone's behavior in contrast to the precipitous anger produced by someone's abrupt and obvious actions.

The vertical progression of self-identity is a reflection of gross human brain anatomy in which three major components of the increasingly complex brain can be identified. *There is a simple hindbrain, a more complex midbrain and a very complex forebrain.* Within the forebrain, there are three major components of the cerebral cortex, two older, less complex, smaller cerebral cortices below but intimately connected to newer, more complex, larger cerebral cortices above. The older cortices are known as the *archipallium* and the *paleopallium*. See figure (6-1). The newer cortices are called the *neocortices* of the cerebral hemispheres. These old and new cortical structures of the forebrain provide us with conscious self-identity.

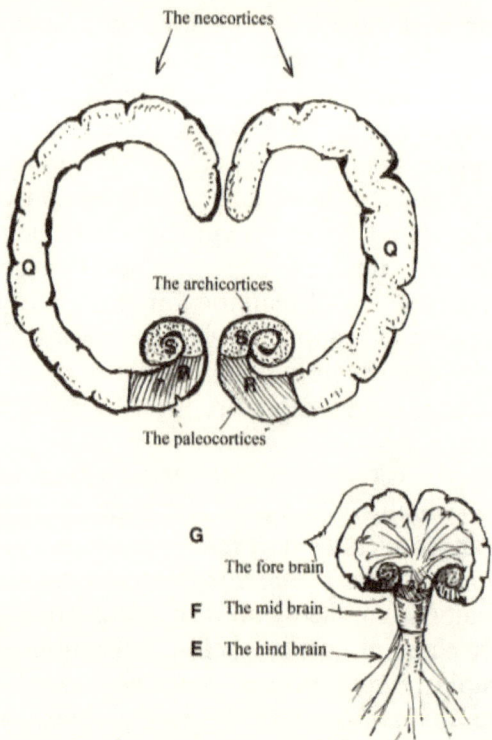

Figure (6-1) A diagram of the three major brain components G, F, E and the three major cortical elements Q, R, S of the brain. The cortex is the outer layer of an organ in the brain; it is the "gray matter". The relative evolutionary status of these three structures is based on considerable comparative anatomical, phylogenetic and evolutionary science in studies of Kappers, Huber and Crosby.

Vertical stacking and integration of older and newer forms of self-identity follow the evolutionary anatomical description of the vertebrate three-part brain. The self and the brain's physical evolution from older brain components to newer ones, each attached to the other are similar. Like the brain, the self appears to be a single entity but actually has older distributed systems connected to newer ones. Rethinking the self as a dynamic evolutionary neurological process of self-identity for survival is taken heavily from the inspiration of contemporary neuro-scientific research that continues to uncover data which support the theory that *the self is actually the brain, not an offspring of a separate energy we have long thought of as spirituous*. However, there has been and will be a great deal of opposition to such a concept.

The human self has departed from its past but is still connected to it. Each newly evolved higher component has a fixed survival reality of awareness and response, but there are traces of the past in each. These individual strategies are united in the human brain in an integrated way that enables humans to regress into more primitive modes of behavioral personality when the occasion demands it. The most complex element controls the lesser complex. The control is essentially an integrated one in which interactions with lower elements are often fluid in action like the action of an automobile's modern transmission. There are other times, the lower control acts like a horse and buggy jolted into action by the report of a rifle.

This evolutionary model, the most primitive element of who we are and what makes us behave in a certain way, is derived from the reptilian component of the human brain. The behavior that comes from that primitive reptilian cortex called the archipallium, is based on defending a fixed territory with primitive animal behavior of fighting, fleeing, foraging and fornicating. Reptilian behavior also has the territorial characteristic that regards all others of its kind therein as a threat to its survival. It doesn't matter if it is the mate, other males or offspring; they are kept in a rigid hierarchical control.

This is the hard core of the self that provides the foundation of our survival and indeed the human personality. The reptile's formula for success continues in all vertebrate animals and ends up as our very own. In the evolution of other animals considered more advanced than the reptile, it is still there but modified by more complicated behavior. It is difficult for many to consider human behavior has anything to do with reptiles, but the influence is there to be appreciated with a little investigation. Credit must be given to those thinkers who established this rather brave assumption about our reptilian cousins.

With due respect to those distant thinkers who wondered about such an inhuman linage, the concept of an evolutionary kind of a human mind-brain was resurrected by Paul D. MacLean when he popularized the concept as the "Triune Brain". It included in addition to the reptile's participation in our mind's behavior, the paleo-mammalian and neo-mammalian components. These three components of the human self appeared to him as a "neuro-chassis", something neuro-anatomical upon which to pin the mind. He was different from Freud who theorized about the mind's parts without hard evidence. MacLean verified anatomically what he believed would reunite the ancient separation of mind and brain. In modern humans, the neuro-chassis of the self in my concept includes more than a triune breakdown of parts because it elaborates on the brain's hemispheric anatomy that provides for the part human evolution played in our modern self-identity. In descending order, there are five significant parts that make up the layers of distributed neuron layers of the self:

D-L. Left cerebral cortex
      Left Neopallium
      Genus Homo self-identity

D-R. Right cerebral cortex
      Right Neopallium
      Anthropoid self-identity

C. The Limbic System, Broca's brain
    The Paleopallium that includes the late Rhinal cortex
    Paleomammalian self-identity

B. The R Complex
    The Diencephalon and early Rhinal cortex
    Reptilian self-identity

A. The lower brain stem
    The mid and hind brain
    Pre-reptilian self-identity

(See figure 6-2.)

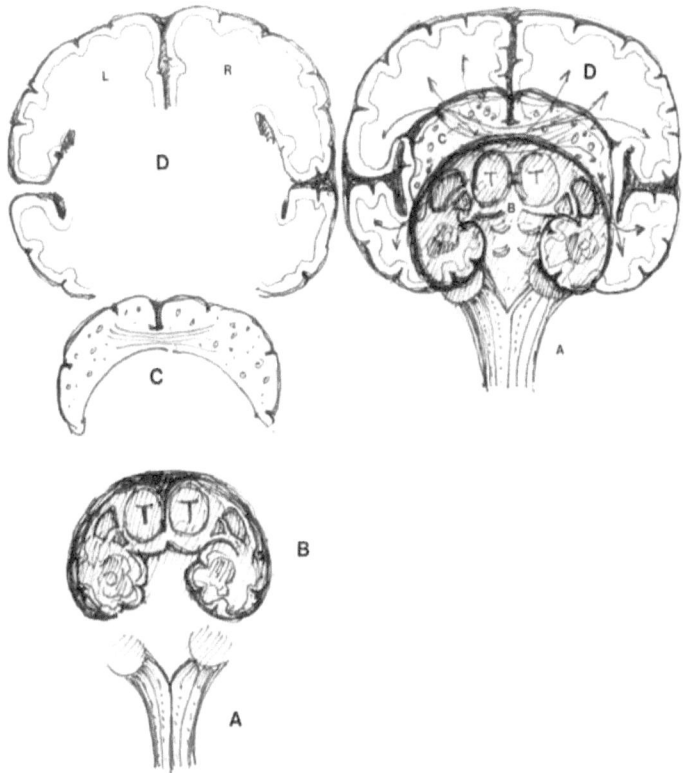

Figure (6-2) A layout of the fundamental layers of self-identity corresponding to the anatomical components of each, beginning with the most complex and ending with the simplest. Each layer of the self is diagrammatically represented as an ascending, larger, more complex interacting neuronal function, called a distributed system of self-identity. (A) The brain stem; Pre-reptilian self-identity. (B) The Diencephalon with the basal ganglia, the thalamus, the hypothalamus and the early rhinal cortical system; Reptilian self-identity. (C) The Limbic system or paleomammalian cortex of the rhinal system. (D-R) The right cerebral hemisphere; Anthropoid self-identity. (D-L) The left cerebral hemisphere; Genus Homo self-identity. In early humans, the right cerebral hemisphere was actually their first intellect and sense of self. Its symbolic nature has continued to evolve in humans, but with respect to self-identity, it remains the legacy of anthropoids and children.

To understand the increasing complexity of the components of the self, evolving from the simple to complex, the appreciation of the cellular contents of the gross anatomical parts is necessary. The basic cell of the brain is the *neuron*. How it functions in the process of human behavior has long been known as first simple and then more complex neuron directed stimulus and response mechanisms. The most simplistic mechanism is called the "spinal reflex" by neuro-physiologists.

This basic mechanism of the nervous system was discovered in 1811 by the English surgeon, Sir Charles Bell. He determined that the nerve cell fibers of the spinal cord were divided by function into two distinct types, the fiber of nerves coming into the brain and the fibers leaving the brain. Eleven years later, a French physiologist, Francois Magendie, not knowing of Bell's work, independently made the same discovery. The knowledge that half of the spinal nerve cells sent impulses *into* the nervous system and the other half sent impulses *out* made intelligible the basic structure of the central nervous system. (And, indeed, it provides the basic understanding of the vertical organization of the self.) See figure (6-3).

As the central nervous system evolved in vertebrates, there was a greater complexity. There was an increased number of neurons involved in what once was a simple process. More neurons were involved in the sensory information coming in and more were involved in understanding the information and sending out appropriate motor action. The nervous system went from simple reflex activity to larger units known as ganglions and eventually to lobes and finally to cortical layers of larger human brains. The self follows the same evolution. What we call the "personality" or "psyche" is organized no differently.

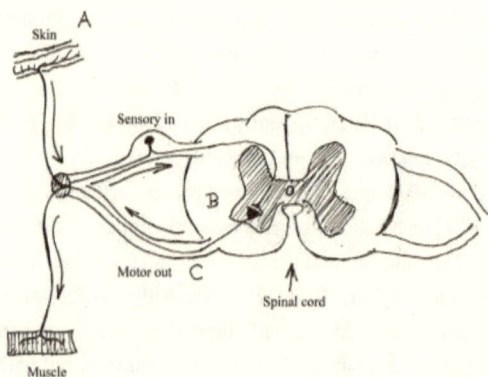

Fig, (6-3) The fundamental organization of the nervous system. Sensations from A are conducted by an afferent sensory neuron to junction B, the synapse, and a second neuron C conducts an efferent motor impulse to a motor unit.

Once again referring to the outline and figure (6-2) of the five elements of the neuro-chassis we will concern ourselves with the four of those vertical layers appreciated as the intellect and the emotions. This simple division of the self can be stimulated by means of the five senses, but in the modern human, survival depends primarily upon symbolic communication, the visual system and the auditory system which are most important and most developed. Because the layers of the self have progressively more evolved neuron complexity, each layer perceives objects in the environment in different ways. With respect to one human perceiving another human, this difference is especially true. The different perceptions of each cortical layer of the self can interpret the same object as dissimilar even though the layers of cortical neurons that represent different layers of the self utilize the same sense organ. We realize that a perception is a more complicated sensory function of the brain than just a sensation because there has been a memory of the object from the various senses in addition to the sensory system directly involved in the perception. Those memories have definite evolutionary characteristics of other kinds of animals and early humans.

As an example, it can be understood that a female of the human species may be regarded in several different ways during a given perception. Let's say that Bob looks up from his desk at a new female candidate for a job as his secretary. What different perceptions are possible with several layers of neurons that make up his diverse self-identity? One, he sees an individual hopefully with qualifications that will fulfill his needs as a secretary, a professional person. Two, he sees a female that is very attractive from the cultural standards of being a "sex object, a possible sexual companion". Three, he sees a potential friend that might enjoy working with him in his unique profession. Four, he might see an enemy who reminds him of his aunt Helen who once in his childhood beat the dickens out of him for some minor indiscretion. As time passes and more information is acquired from the female object by means of increased stimulation and response with her, one layer may become more stimulated than the others and that layer of the self may well bring about an obvious behavior typical of that layer.

For those readers who are unfamiliar with the neuron theory of how these cells in the brain function, to help understand, we can simplify what neurons do in terms of a simple stimulus and a response process similar to the example above. From a psychological perspective we can observe a behavior of an animal by stimulating it in a certain way and seeing what effect that stimulation has on the animal's behavior. In a similar manner we can do the same experiment but in microscopic terms based on how neurons function under the same circumstances. In a brief review of neuron mechanics, neurons are cells of the nervous system that individually or in groups can be stimulated to cause a certain nervous system cellular response. Recall it was described how early neuroanatomists discovered that nerve fibers of certain neurons brought information into the core of the nervous system and certain neurons expressed a response to that stimulation. In figure (6-4), a sensory neuron cell is diagrammed with its major components labeled as: 1) the sensory ending, 2) the axon leading to 3) the cell body from which 4) the dendrite comes in contact with the cell body of a motor neuron at 5) the synapse of the two basic neuron types, 6) the axon of the motor neuron that joins to 7) some form of motor structure usually a muscle fiber or glandular structure. In figure (6-5), a sensory neuron is diagrammed to show that it can have more than one dendrite that does something besides actively synapse with a motor neuron. These other dendrites are capable of inhibiting a different synapse elsewhere and there are still others that can inhibit those dendrites that are inhibiting a synapse.

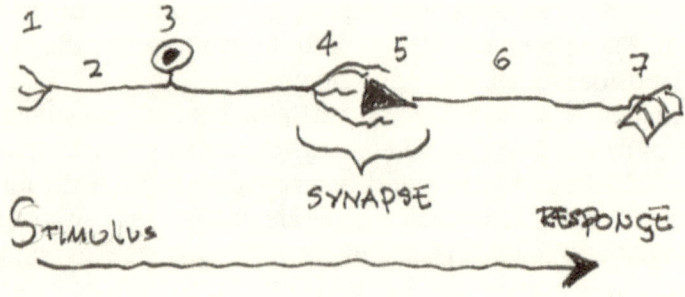

Figure (6-4) Diagram of the synapse between a sensory and a motor neuron.

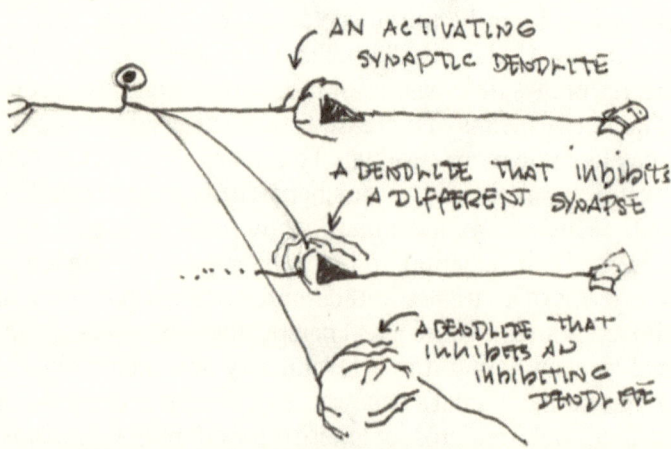

Figure (6-5) A Diagram of various dendrite functions.

Each cortical brain structure with its different mentality has these elements within its cellular makeup. The multiple functions of sensory dendrites are necessary to explain the activation of one specific cortex and the inhibition of a competing cortex. The great number of these competing units provides a modulation of their individual behavior either damping one while enhancing the other depending upon the particular strength of the stimulus acting on the sensory endings.

In the normal human of a modern society, it will be further appreciated that the left word symbolic brain's outer cortex of reason acts as the primary mediator of the needs of the individual's total sense of self. It's the part of the central nervous system that results in talking and thinking behavior. It is also the agent that attempts to express what is going on in the entire central nervous system and it will most often take the most pacific means of survival by talking itself out of trouble. The "mind" as it is otherwise known, also must be alert to stimulation from others who have less than the highest form of intellectual competitiveness and use more primitive forms of reasoning and emotional means of survival. Of course, it is fundamentally important for survival of a normal individual to regress into lower emotional survival behavior when the need calls for it.

In a pacific environment, vertical as well as horizontal integration of the human self involves a neuron driven state of equilibrium between the intellect on the left and the right visually oriented most evolved cerebral cortex and the lower emotions that are aligned with it. Otherwise said, it occurs when the body language of a person agrees with the auditory language of that person. There is disequilibrium when body language doesn't agree with auditory language wherein what the emotions are "feeling" is discordant with what is being said. When the intellectual mind-states and the emotional mind-states of the brain are in equilibrium they are in a static agreement or at rest. At rest, they are in a state of readiness to be stimulated. Stimulation of any one or more of the brain's vertical (and later to be explained, horizontal progressively more complex layers) can cause a state of disequilibrium.

For example, let us examine what happens when the equilibrium between the two basic emotions is disrupted by stimulation of one of them. In figure (6-6), the R (reptilian) layer of the basic emotions of fear and anger, the most primitive human layer, is shown to be in equilibrium with the next higher level of the basic emotions, PM (paleo-mammalian or limbic) layer, the emotions of love and mating. (This concept should be compared to the Papez theory of the emotions' neuro-circuitry.) The vertical electro chemical equilibrium between these two neuron pools is brought by an equal amount of reciprocal inhibition of each layer by the other. Equilibrium of the two systems is in a "steady state" of inaction, ready for action. This is caused by the inhibitory dendrites of both systems equally acting on each others' synaptic junctions joined to their specific motor neurons.

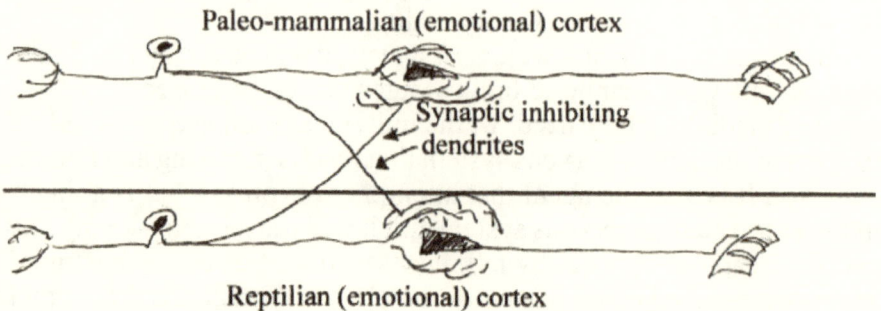

Figure (6-6) A diagram of an equilibrium of the two emotional systems, Reptilian and Paleo-mammalian, brought about by a resting reciprocal inhibition of both layers by synaptic inhibiting dendrites.

When the R (reptilian) emotions are stimulated by an appropriate stimulus, an angry sound, for example, the equilibrium is disrupted between the two layers wherein the stimulated sensory axons of R cause microscopic activation of its motor neurons. This stimulus simultaneously activates the sensory neurons' specific inhibitory dendrites of the PM neuron pool. The state of disequilibrium is shown in figure (6-7). Here the inhibition of PM by R takes place as more neurons of R are stimulated for action and concurrently inhibit more inhibitory dendrites of the PM neuron pool. We refer this as a process of neuron recruitment. It reaches a mesoscopic level of neuron pool excitation as defined by Freeman. We would subjectively appreciate this shift as an inner feeling of modest discomfort with what was happening: "I was beginning to feel things weren't going to be pleasant." With still greater stimulation of R it becomes entirely free of inhibition from PM because PM inhibitory neurons are totally inhibited. This refers to a macroscopic threshold and the motor neurons of action of this assemblage are activated for a specific behavior of fight or flight.

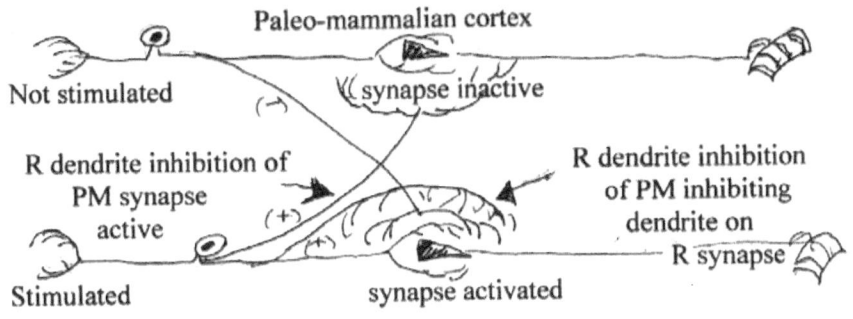

Figure (6-7) A diagram of a shift in equilibrium to disequilibrium of two systems after stimulation of one, R causes inhibition of the other's PM inhibition of R.

In this vertical and horizontal integration of the self that involves the intellects and the emotions, we should remember Freud was very much interested in behavior that he characterized as suppression and regression. It is likely that he did not appreciate these behaviors were driven by populations of different layers of cortical neurons that interacted by a reciprocal inhibiting integration. As Lee pointed out, "Each level of the self modifies the activities of the layer just beneath it." Freeman describes the situation in his research as a homeostatic neuronal feedback which serves to keep things in a steady state when not being stimulated.

To demonstrate this process further, when you are on the phone with someone, you have no way of seeing what is happening with either the visual systems of Reptilian cortex or Paleomammalian cortex. As your conversation proceeds in the direction of stimulation of R rather than PM, you would appreciate a slow burning anger rising in you that would be progressively expressed in angry sounding words as well as words and combinations of words that mean anger. If the conversation continues in that direction, you would end up shouting words and then loud obscenities at the person on the other end of the line and you might well react with a total body response and slam down the receiver. Therefore, any one or a combination of the senses can activate a layer of human self-identity and by means of a reciprocal vertical inhibition of each other's synaptic junctions, one system can be liberated for action or two systems can be activated with a combined response of each.

Let us now examine what happens when the left auditory sensory cortex receives a mixed message wherein the emotional neuron pool for fight or flight is stimulated by angry or frightening word symbols, but the prosody, the emotional sounds of the words, are spoken softly and with affection, thereby stimulating the emotional neuron pool for attraction. For example, if I said, "I want to kill you." in a soft, seductive voice, two emotional layers would be stimulated, but in an antagonistic way. The words mean one thing; the way they are spoken means another. In this situation, both R and PM neuron pools are stimulated. The R pool is stimulated by the meaning of the words and the PM pool is contrarily stimulated by the sound of the words; the sounds of the words are seductive and comforting. In this case, an individual will not know exactly how to feel or respond to the mixed stimulus. It will only be obvious when the sounds of the words and the words themselves are both directed to either the R or the PM pool.

In this regard, it is important to understand that angry sounds are the appropriate stimulus for the reptilian layer of the emotions just as auditory symbols of angry thoughts are appropriate. Epithets and swear words are symbolic examples as well as the statement: "I hate you". The sounds and specific words that intend fear and anger activate the reptilian, the old mammalian, and the anthropoid emotional cortex in two ways. First, the "sound" goes directly to the emotional layers and second, "the word symbol of fear or anger" has to be learned by the auditory-word symbolic sensory cortex of Wernicke and its associated auditory motor cortex. This learning is a conditioning process between the word symbol and the emotional state. In this context, the word can stimulate the lower emotional levels of self almost as easily as the environment or the real stimulus of fear or anger are able to do. Consequently, with respect to the auditory system, we are more often stimulated at the emotional layers with both the words and how the words sound. They are more often synergistic, not antagonistic. See figure (6-8).

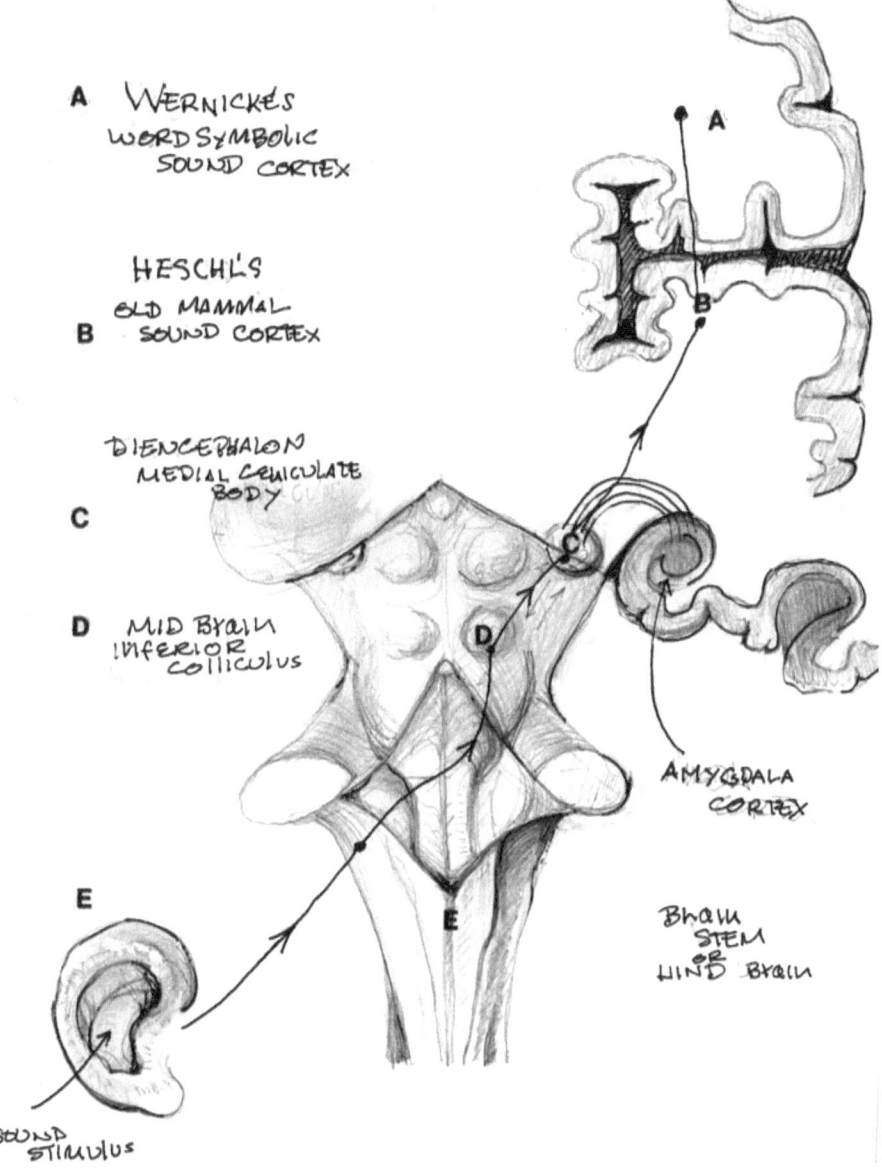

A WERNICKE'S
WORD SYMBOLIC
SOUND CORTEX

B HESCHL'S
OLD MAMMAL
SOUND CORTEX

C DIENCEPHALON
MEDIAL GENICULATE
BODY

D MID BRAIN
INFERIOR
COLLICULUS

E

AMYGDALA
CORTEX

BRAIN
STEM
OR
HIND BRAIN

SOUND
STIMULUS

Figure (6-8) The hypothetical vertical flow of an auditory stimulus that consists of both angry sounds and words which stimulate the reptilian cortex, the paleomammalian cortex and Wernicke's auditory symbolic cortex.

Referring to figure (6-8), one can trace the stations on the trip the stimulus passes through beginning in the hind brain (the medulla oblongata) at (E), then to the inferior colliculus of the mid brain at (D), the startle level of awareness. Then from the startle station, the stimulus travels upward to the diencephalon's medial geniculate body, the reptilian level of self-identity at (C). Here it passes through the thalamus and the connections to the amygdaloid cortex that produces the behavior of fight or flight and the primitive emotions of fear and anger. The stimulus continues vertically (actually rostrally) upward to Heschl's primary auditory cortex at (B), the transverse temporal gyrus of the temporal lobe which recognizes more variations of fearful and angry sounds as well as other pacific, pleasant sounds that are typical for old and new mammals. Finally the sound stimulus proceeds to the neocortex only on the left cerebral side at (A), Wernicke's word symbolic cortex that has come to recognize words and thoughts. This final station would possess only a robotic appreciation of words or thoughts if they were not influenced, colored and modified by the lower emotional layers.

Modulated neuronal interaction of self-identity layers can be explained in another way by what neurologists have found to occur in walking which requires the reciprocal inhibition of certain muscle groups by others. Certain groups of muscles stop working while other groups are working. When we lift a leg to begin walking the muscles that return the leg to the ground must be inhibited. The inhibition must also be modulated or regulated to achieve a smooth transition from one muscle action to the other. We can suddenly lift a leg in a jerk of movement or we can walk slowly or run rapidly. The actions of our self-identities behave in the same manner.

The Distributed Systems of Vertical Self-Identity

At the top of the self-identity system of the brain is:

A. Genus Homo Self-Identity—*the auditory symbolic level of neurons primarily located in the left auditory language areas of the left neocortex; the mind with its voice. See figure (6-9).*

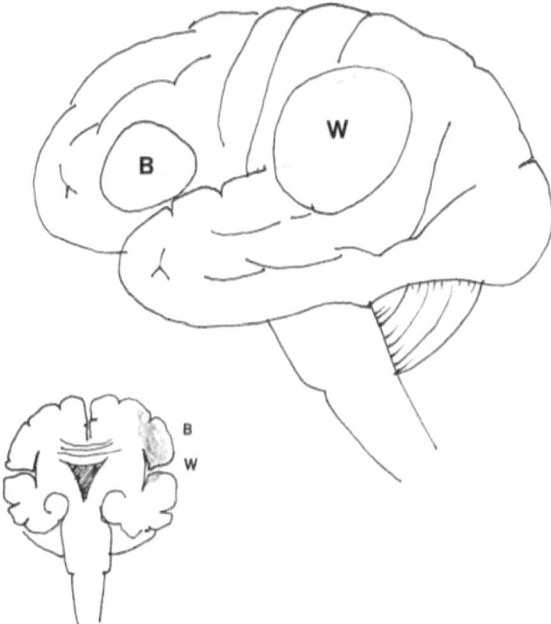

Figure (6-9) The most evolved vertical element of self-identity for most humans is a portion of the left cerebral hemisphere at (B) and (W). It is a cortical neuron assemblage specific for communication with sound symbols internally in the process of thinking, or externally with others who know the meaning of the sound symbols. (W) represents Wernicke's sensory arm of the system and (B) represents Broca's motor arm of the system.

The most complex element of self-identity and all other lower levels function within the fundamental organization of Bell's original discovery of nerve cells. Language, either spoken, in thoughts, or communicated otherwise comes in and reactive language information goes out. This is the most complex level of self-identity in which word symbols act as sensory input to the brain and word symbols act as motor output from the brain. Word symbols have provided Homo Sapiens a greater advantage for survival than other animals. Some symbols provide man with a greater ability, far beyond the capacity of other animals, to know what is coming without actually experiencing it.* With symbols, Egyptian engineers could measure heavy limestone blocks without taking them to the top of the pyramid and back again to see if they would fit in place. This layer

---

*   Many animals, however, are equipped to sense natural catastrophes well ahead of humans without access to scientific information.

of self-identity also provides humans with an ability to think in word symbols which provide ideas and concepts that often have not been proved with verification by the primary senses but more often than not, are later shown to be so. Thinking in its highest form most importantly allows for individual action without an abnormal dependence on others.

Within this layer of the hierarchical self-identity system are less effective survival forms of auditory symbolic communication. These older, less efficient means of thinking reflect the now evolved older language capabilities of our human ancestors. These forms are the ancient human obligations to do exactly what others tell a person to do, to say exactly what others have told a person to say. They include the early communication with symbols to believe what others have told them to believe and to think in dependent terms of: "You made me do it." or "See what you made me do." R.D. Laing has described how a personality is formed during childhood because of the great suggestibility of language at that period. When Mom calls daughter a "bad girl", the child far too often assumes that character.

Modern thinking of most western humans continues to have remnants of older forms of thinking. Mature humans pass through and absorb, but do not discard primitive ways of thinking. They revert back to these forms when there is trouble that can't be managed.* Theodor Reik provides ample evidence that mental illness is characterized by primitive thinking processes from the mystical-magical, fantastic-omnipotent and early religious history of man's thinking. Saying it makes it real; wishing it makes it happen; doing a ritualistic, unrelated thing could make something wished for happen; thinking about an act to oneself was as real as the actual observable act. These primitive ways of thinking, once thought to be characteristics of neurotics and psychotics, in reality, are part of every human's thinking process but they have been subverted and are under the control of newer ways of thinking.

Ancient language thinking processes are appropriate during the acquisition of language in children learning to think. Children can imagine an almost real mental transformation of themselves into machines, animals and other humans. With further mind development, they pass through this stage as well as others to become relatively rational. As normal adults, they become aware only fleetingly of wishes and fantasies.

Recent psychoanalytic observations of Berne appreciate that most humans under certain stresses resort to *child* or *childlike-parent* behaviors.

---

* Early psychoanalytical investigation that uncovered these old forms of thinking led to the belief they were only neurotic processes of mentally ill individuals.

At times, those with a fully developed sense of self, as well as neurotics and psychotics, regress to use older forms of thinking to manage the stresses. More often than not, immature thinking is the result of inadequate development of independent thought. The lack of independent thinking causes dependency states in which individuals cannot fully care for themselves as members of society. Those with over-dependency are unable to compete with independent thinkers.

Below the highest self-identity layer of the brain is:

B. Primate self-identity—*the visually oriented neurons characteristic of anthropoid behavior located primarily in the right temporal-parietal and occipital cortices of the right neocortex. See figure 6-10.*

The brain, as most of us appreciate, evolved into two large cortical hemispheres that don't show any vertical linearity of self-identity. Regardless, in the modern human, the left auditory symbolic cortex is dominant over the right visual cortex. As pointed out in the chapter on simian self-identity, in some humans, the dominance of the auditory cortex is incomplete and those individuals exhibit behavior in which the vision-silent-emotional right cortical part of the self is in control. These are the individuals who in development do not fully join what they say and what they do. This retarded development isn't a dissociation of mind and body, but an incomplete neurological control of the right hemisphere by the left. Individuals with the monkey-emotional-child self of the right hemisphere in control, use words but don't live up to them. Individuals, for the most part in control of their actions with their left hemisphere, can often reveal the influence of the right hemisphere in what they say in the form of Freudian slips of the tongue, the blocking of names, double and triple entendres and conversations with subtexts and secondary agendas of emotionally charged child-like behavior.

This right hemispheric level of self-identity expresses behavior primarily in prosematics, otherwise known as body language, and in highly developed facial expressions. This part of the self is silent, non-verbal. It solves survival problems, for the most part, by body acts and emotional behavior. It is visible behavior that may or may not be witnessed by others. This self-identity can be out of sync with the auditory symbolic self. It may actually contradict what is being said. It can also guide an observer to know that talking is not succeeding and the individual is closer to emotional acts of the body. In the Western human, this part of self-identity is the doppelganger, the unknown, silent side of the individual. It is also the part of the self that provides new ideas with visual images, which may include diagrams, formulas, and pictures. This visual brain is yoked to the auditory brain by neurons in the occipital cortex to produce written symbols of verbal language primarily on the left, but it also provides a stream of neurons to the motor cortex on the right that prepares a mechanism for a visual moving stimulus of a dancer, for example, to be mimicked by another person watching the dancer. While this layer is the fundamental basis of visually symbolic intelligence gained through visual intuition and imagination that compliment auditory symbolic intelligence, it also can cause regressive survival behaviors in which groups are involved. The ancestral origins of simian behavior of this sort provide the strength of multiple individuals in riots, gangbangs and the sangfroid of men in battle. When control by the more advanced, linear thinking, auditory hemisphere falters in command of the whole self, the visual brain behaves as a "fubar". It drops things, forgets to do things, can't keep focused on tasks and disrupts human activities with child-like attention deficits and passive-aggressive behavior. In its most evolved development, the right visually oriented hemisphere has created the philosophies of Eastern cultures and it has also provided the genius of artistic expression.

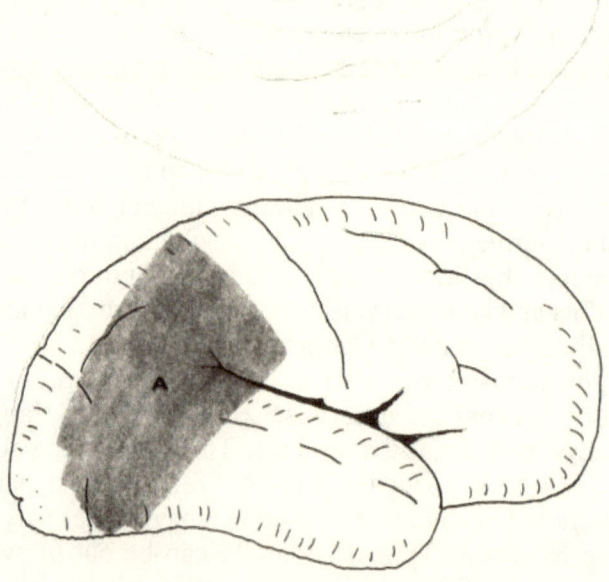

Figure (6-10) The primate vertical element of self-identity is a portion of the right cerebral hemisphere. It is a cortical neuron assemblage that involves visual communication by body language, sign language and facial expression.

At a lower level of the brain is:

C. Paleomammalian self-identity—*the neurons of the self-identity system that express the behavior of old mammals in family groups and pair bonds. See figure (6-11).*

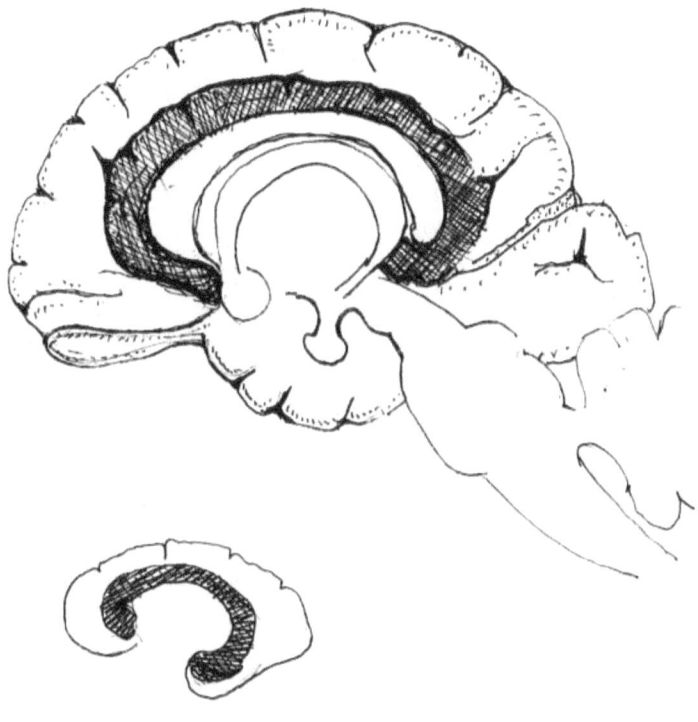

Broca's
Limbic lobe

Figure (6-11): A schematic of the paleomammalian level of human self-identity. Anatomically it consists of a major part of Broca's limbic lobe, but does not include the hippocampi and the amygdalae. These two elements considered by MacLean to be a part of the limbic lobe have always been considered elements of the archipallium or the oldest human cortex that preceded the brains of mammals.

Anatomists have had a conflicting understanding of this part of the lower brain of humans. In the nineteenth century, Broca understood that the neocortex was divided into a neopallium and a paleopallium; the latter he called the limbic lobe that was the brain responsible for smell derived behavior typical of old mammals. The smaller hidden paleopallium evolved prior to the larger neopallium or neocortex, *but the archipallium evolved before both*. Broca included the archipallium as part of the limbic lobe. Earlier anatomists identified a part of what Broca considered to be part of the limbic lobe as just the gyrus fornicatus and the gyrus cinguli, but not part of any limbic lobe as Broca envisioned it. Yet they appreciated that the gyrus fornicatus cortex under the neocortex was related to sexual activity in mammals. Later in the 1950's, neuro-anatomists rejected the concept of Broca's limbic lobe. However, in the 1960's, MacLean included Broca's concept of a limbic system of neurons in a model of his own.

My concept, based on evolutionary anatomical evidence, considers the paleo-mammalian system of human self-identity to include the gyrus fornicatus and gyrus cinguli of Broca's limbic lobe, but does not include the amygdalae and hippocampi of MacLean's model.

Deeper yet in the human brain is:

D. Reptilian self-identity—*the neurons that make up the reptilian system of human self-identity. This system expresses the behavior of reptiles with autocratic control of territory, mates and hierarchical rivals. These neurons are primarily located in the diencephalon of the forebrain. These neurons provide the archicortex or archipallium with the fundamental responses we refer to as instincts. See figure (6-12).*

In 1928, Bard, the authority of his day, identified the major emotions of anger and fear. They are our primal emotions for survival. This survival core sense of self continues to influence all other systems of self in a relatively positive sense as we, in modern societies, become more pacific, yet in a negative sense as many of us fail developmentally to achieve an appropriate inhibition of fear and anger and the need to dominate others.

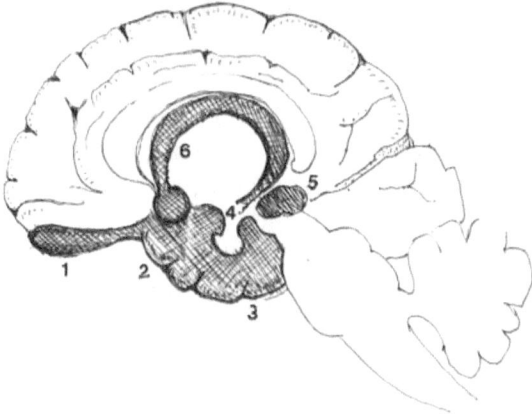

Figure (6-12) The reptilian component of human self-identity anatomically consists of (1) the olfactory bulb (2) the paired amgydalae and (3) paired hippocampi (4) the hypothalamus (5) the paired basal ganglia (6) the fornix.

Some neurologists claim the limbic system is responsible for both love, anger and fear emotions. Furthermore, MacLean's anatomical concept of the reptilian brain system in man does not include key areas that provide for basic reptilian behavior. MacLean's diagrams place vital reptilian behavior in the limbic lobe of Broca. I propose that the reptilian component must include the amygdalae and the hippocampi because these archicortical systems preceded in evolution those typical of mammals. Referring to figure (6-13), it can be appreciated that each newly evolved brain component becomes part of a newer one.

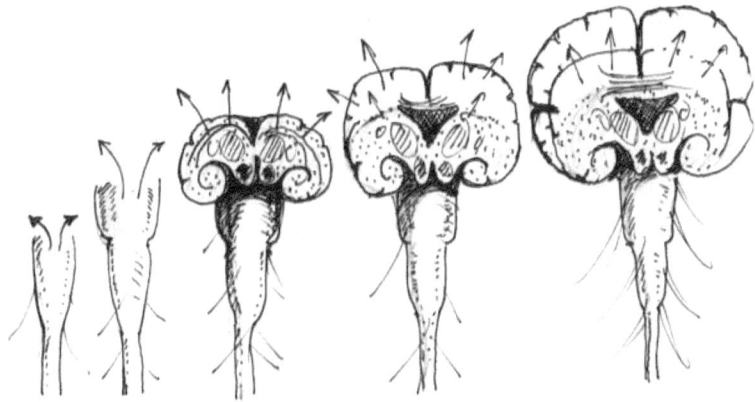

Figure (6-13) A schematic appreciation of older brain parts being assimilated into newer ones.

MacLean did not include the olfactory bulb and its archicortical elements as part of the reptilian brain component. The olfactory system was well in place in other earlier vertebrates such as fishes and sharks. The vertebrate phylum is of enormous antiquity and stems from the primitive agnatha or jawless pre-fishes. Living in a totally watery environment, early vertebrates had a primary sense of being separate from the environment by means of a sensory system that could pick up molecular chemical traces of prey, mates and predators at great distances. This chemical sensory system of their prime identity drove their behavior in water and somewhat confusingly is referred to as their "olfactory system". The confusion is derived from our limited appreciation that the olfactory system of smell in mammals including ourselves, occurs only in the environment of gaseous matter we call air. Olfaction began in water and evolved with amphibians, reptiles and mammals to include the air environment. For all of vertebrate history until the appearance of the neo-mammals, the simians, the principal sense of self was olfactory, first for sensations in water, then a combination of water and air and then only in air.

When Broca defined the limbic lobe in the nineteenth century, it was initially believed that its smell sensory dependent character was typical of old mammals solely. What came into common acceptance failed to take into account that "the smell brain" of Broca with its rhinal systems, was derived from reptiles. The knowledge that the olfactory system of reptiles evolved from the chemical senses of earlier vertebrates in water was overlooked. Smell sense in fishes and sharks was chemical in a water-soluble environment. The chemical sense, thought to be the oldest sensory system known, was available to vertebrate life in salt water long before mammals appeared. As amphibians and reptiles emerged from their saline environment and began to live on land this sense evolved to recognize chemicals in air. This new sense of smell was a transformed, older one in which the reptile sensed the world with a mixed form of the old sense and the newer one.

The olfactory sense of the reptile is highly unique. It is accomplished by means of detecting chemicals in the air with a forked tongue that senses air molecules and presents them to the roof of its mouth where a structure known as *Jacobson's organ* has evolved. The essential evolutionary issue is that these creatures have retained fish chemo-receptors on the roofs of their mouths. This fact is evidence of primitive olfaction in transition characterized by the development of *Jacobson's organ* and a long forked tongue which could be projected into the air. In an accommodation between the watery world of fishes and land-bound mammals, the reptile and the amphibian have developed a smell system that utilizes the tongue.

There is justification, therefore, to include the primitive rhinal system as a fundamental element of the reptilian nervous system. The reptilian cortex is recapitulated in humans in the amygdalae and the adjacent hippocampi. These two primitive cortical structures have long been considered as part of the rhinal system of mammals, but they are best identified as elements of the brain of reptiles. Again, it is important to remember that removal of the amygdalae, from almost all animals, rids them of their aggressive reptilian behavior.

From an evolved origin, there is a basic order to everyone's self-identity and while we are different, we all have elements in common. We humans all have different faces, but faces in common. We all have different fingerprints but prints in common; the same goes for the anatomy of our irises, our retinal vasculature and our DNA. However, each whole self-identity must develop from birth within a critical fixed period. The development is brought about by other humans of a specific cultural environment in a process of entraining or triggering. The genetic material within sensory neurons of the brain essentially must assimilate external human-environmental stimuli to become a complete self in a fixed time.

The great variety of human self-identity is a result of the varied development brought about by those that provide the development. While the chassis is genetically provided, it is not fixed in our character at birth. It must be stimulated and regulated to develop fully. Neuroscientists are aware that at birth there are "committed" parts of the human brain for specific motor and sensory functions. Committed means that those areas are ready to do specific tasks, but they need development and integration with other cortical brain elements to become fully active. In essence, something must be added to the chassis to make it run like a modern human.

In this regard, ophthalmologists appreciate that at birth the occipital cortex is committed to the visual system but is not fully developed. At birth, the vision of a newborn is hardly 20/20 and must be stimulated to develop during the first six years of life to achieve a high degree of efficiency. Otherwise, it remains at the level of the reptile's acuity. If either eye is not stimulated by use during the first six years, a stunting called "amblyopia" will occur.

In a similar manner, the older components of self are committed to their interactive functions but must develop and integrate with other newer brain systems of the self. The human brain at birth has been compared to a *tabula rasa* but is much more like a seed waiting for the right seasonal environment in which to grow. The infant-self starts the process of a vertical development and integration, again like a seed beginning to sprout.

This vertical development and integration have to do with genetically scheduled traffic between the evolved components. The developing self in each newborn infant must recapitulate the evolution of neurons of the species of mankind to acquire a full complexity of behavior necessary for survival. There is no catapult propulsion to becoming human with full self-identity. Yet, it is a sequential process faster than the eye can see. If passengers are at the airport in a specific stage of development no matter in what shape of preparedness they are for departure, they must get on the plane. A child may have acquired a distorted emotional self-identity when the plane of auditory language self-identity is ready for take off. No matter what the state the child's emotional self-identity is, the child must board the plane of developing language.

In the highly evolved human brain nothing has been lost. The primitive neuron reflex circuit still exists in the visual system. For example, the eye responds by constriction to a small stimulus of light even though vision has more complex functions. The increasing complexity of input and output of the spinal reflex can be explained neurologically if one considers the hierarchical organization of brain motor systems in vertebrates. After studying motor derangements associated with seizures, the nineteenth century English neurologist, John Hughlings Jackson established that: "In evolution there had been a progression from automatic toward purposive movements and this is reflected in the nervous system in the control of automatic movements by lower levels of the brain and purposive movements by higher levels of the brain and that this control can be either excitatory or inhibitory. When upper level function is interrupted or destroyed by disease, lower centers are released from higher control and result often in hyperactivity."

Contemporary observations of brain damaged children by Delacato also demonstrate this classic organization. When higher levels of neurological function fail, the next lower level becomes dominant. There is similar evidence of this increasing complexity of neurological function found in sensory systems of the brain. The process is also readily appreciated from past observation of emotions. Cannon and Bard have found that removing the forebrain cortex of cats, but leaving the hypothalamus caused the animals to be extremely irritable, triggered into rage at the slightest provocation. Further studies have confirmed their observations, that when the transaction of monkey brains occurred just below the hypothalamus the rage response was lost.

These historical neurological observations can be applied to the system of self as it is vertically related in progressive elements of complexity from below upwards. The similar mechanisms of animal behavior to human emotional behavior help explain why certain humans act like reptiles, old mammals and early hominids. They look human and talk a good game, but their very essence is related to a stunting in development of their vertical self-identity.

Once more intricate components of the brain with their complex self-identity characteristics evolved, a process of integration occurred to unite larger distributed systems with more primitive systems of the self. *The primary neuronal element of vertical integration is a reciprocal inhibition of lower parts by higher ones.*

Less complex lower elements of self-identity are kept under control by higher layers. If higher layers are damaged or do not develop, lower layers of self-identity are unusually hyperactive and are in control just as Jackson and Delacato observed with derangement of motor systems of the brain. In the normal human that has developed a sense of self fully, his less modern senses of self are kept under inhibition by higher centers until their expression is appropriate. No ablation experiments are necessary in those individuals who have not developed a complete sense of self. Their basic behavior is a life-long experiment in which they are uninhibited humans all too ready to be enraged.

In the human, the cortical layers that inhibitory impulses must pass through act as different mentalities. The most complex provides a sensory awareness that we like to consider rational-human, the intellectual self. The less complex layers provide a sensory awareness we understand as the emotional-animal self. One emotional-self, which evolved with the paleo-mammalians, nurtures and sustains relationships. The other emotional-self which evolved from the reptiles does just the opposite. Humans are the recipients of four mentalities with a neural ability that provides for a fluid or immediate utilization of combinations of these different selves. The self can be transformed from being "cool" to "hot-headed" with the speed of neuron impulses. It has been brought to light that those humans less fortunate in their full maturation of a human self, either in a less evolved society or as derelicts in our own, control their behavior from a more primitive level of self, mostly emotional. These individuals try to survive with whatever brain tools they have acquired. Conversely, individuals, who are considered to be relatively well developed and in possession of all the mentalities of the nervous system for survival, are able to utilize any one of a combination of these mentalities for survival by a neurological mechanism referred to as a "regressive synaptic response". When thinking and talking elements of our higher self don't have an answer to compete at a high level of rational intelligence, a regression to what was once a routine, old human, way of thinking takes place. If the circumstance can't be managed by this step in regressive action, regression may proceed further to anger-fear responses and eventually to withdrawal.

When language fails, when appeasement fails, the reptilian manifesto of survival comes into action. It's time for fight or flight. Neuron clusters in the distributed cortical systems of the layered self attempt to interact with an appropriateness that is typical of each layer of the self, just as a simple stimulus and response occur in the primitive spinal reflex. When there is not a well-developed appropriate stimulus-response way of surviving within a given layer, a regression to a lower response layer is possible. See figure (6-14). This regressive capability of the nervous system provides safeguards against extinction. As history has shown in cultural and national conflicts in which the participants are of different degrees of evolution, the system of regression is mandatory.

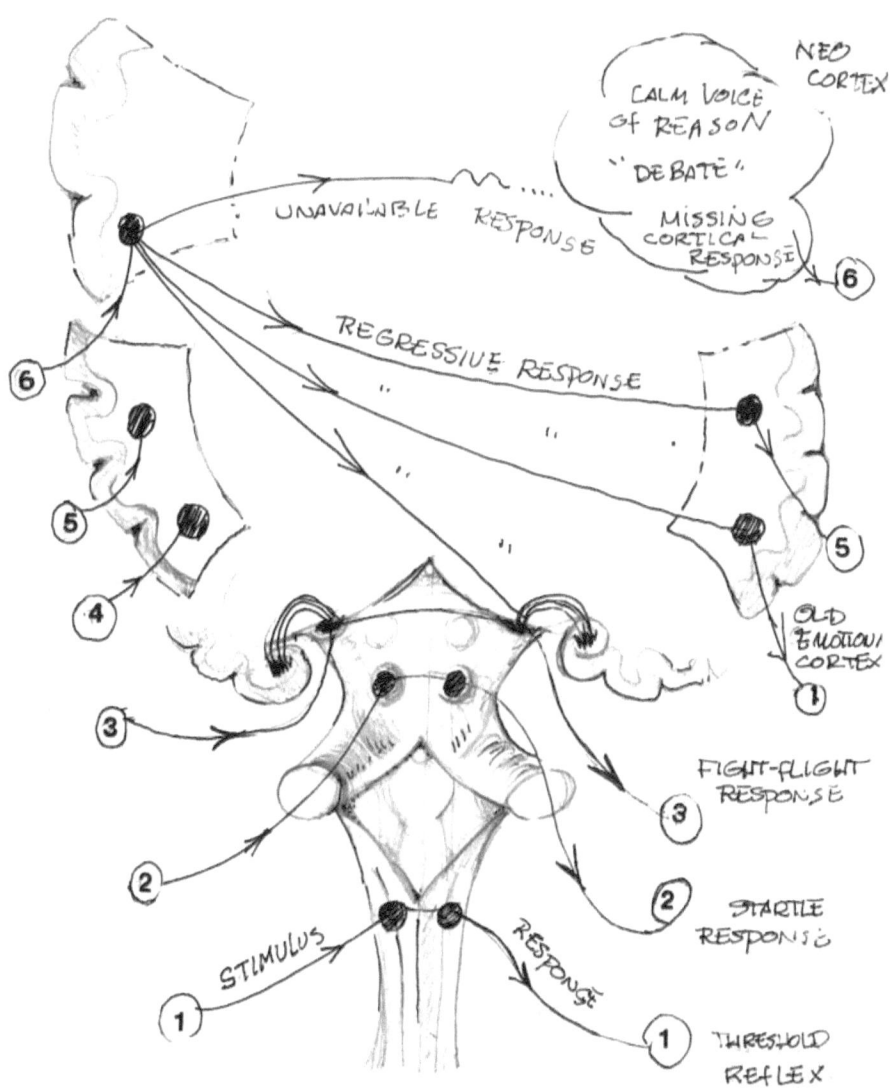

Figure (6-14) A diagram showing the vertical regressive stimulus-response mechanisms of the human nervous system. The cascade of responses is numbered from the most complex @ 6 to the most rudimentary @ 1.

Chapter 7

Horizontal Integration of the Human Self-Identity Components

How the multiple senses interrelate.

In the fall of 1994 Dr. Kaminski was in San Francisco. He was attending a post-graduate meeting to acquire credits towards his state's requirements for licensure to practice medicine. He was there for a second reason in which he would reinvent a misperception he had long held about himself. The national meeting would provide an unpalatable awareness that he wasn't as special as he thought being a specialist entitled him to be. He would again discover he was just another anonymous face in a vast audience of fellows from all across the country. The meeting opened an old narcissistic wound of the burdensome realization—some specialists were more important than others. Being lost in the crowd, it all painfully came back to him. Vast was his specialty consisting of more than seven thousand members and organized in what appeared to be an expression of democratic satisfaction to all. Unfortunately, Kaminski saw it as a very personal dissatisfaction. To him, it was a horizon-less territory that allowed one president and a large executive branch to lord over a herd of followers. He had a badge that identified his membership in the professional society. The badge provided some minimal distinction between him and candidates, foreigners, the drug salesmen, the secretaries, technicians and salespeople, but the badge was bare of brightly colored ribbons that in a casual glance told others the importance of those members that possessed them. He was tired and disappointed at the end of hours of just being an onlooker. He felt he knew as much as those adjusting microphones under bright spotlights, taking applause and receiving honors.

At the end of the day Dr. Kaminski was glad to slip away to a quiet bar. He wanted drinking to do more than savor local wines he remembered from his internship in the Bay Area. He anticipated an anesthesia of his perceived mediocrity. His old pal, Dr. Roger Quigley, who had driven up from Monterrey for no other reason than to see Kaminski joined him. After the first glass produced its euphoric effects and the greetings were over, Kaminski asked his psychiatrist friend what he thought of an article he had been carrying around for this exact occasion. Matters of psychological interest discussed with psychiatrist Quigley, like booze kept his mind away from the gloom of inferiority.

"What the hell is this guy talking about? Read this for me, it's not very long." Dr. Quigley twisted his torso to get a shaft of light coming from a distant window. Waiting, Kaminski let his own eyes entertain him with the passing of attractive female silhouettes.

"This is very strange stuff," Quigley announced, chuckling to his only listener. "Perhaps it's just a case of a kook who thinks he is more than one person, nice example of a split personality." Quigley had just finished a small vignette by a famous Argentinean author, Jorge Luis Borges who had written in an obscure journal that he really felt separated from his mind, but was under the control of his mind that directed his body to do things and took credit for things that he, Borges, had written. Borges revealed a sense of despondency realizing he had to share his life with a mind that directed him around and took credit for everything. At the end of the little piece of self-deprecation, he commented: *"I don't know which of us wrote this."*

"Look at it this way," Quigley continued, "Borges refers to himself as being not out of his mind but separate from it, as if his mind really was just part of him. Usually we think of a mind as the real 'me' up there in our heads. In Borges' case he was in competition with it. He was somehow not just his mind. I say to you: 'I've got this notion in my mind.' It's not much different. I am telling you I am also separate from my mind. I am saying it's a possession of mine in a figurative sense. It's just a way of speaking." On he went, "the word 'mind' when you use it that way is just referring to the whole person and he uses the word 'mind' instead of the word 'I'." Then Quigley hastened to ask, doubting his own explanation, "Could an individual really appreciate that his mind was just one of his brain's parts? Aren't you your mind? How can it be all of you; how can it even be the entire psyche if you can lose it and still appreciate yourself being there? The man is ridiculous, but you know . . . ." Then Quigley placed his upper lip on the rim of his wine glass in a characteristic pose suggesting deep thought. "People keep talking about losing their minds especially when they are becoming deeply schizophrenic; they are still aware of a mind that is separate from them until it is lost. They can still be there and feel it slipping away. Is it more than a figure of speech? Does language usage tell us something else?"

Kaminski became agitated at these bizarre comments. Already, in such a short time, Kaminski thought, Quigley was finding a way to explain his original perplexity about what Borges had written. He joined in, "I feel just like Borges; I am not just my mind because the way I use language tells me it is separate from me. I use the word 'my' to indicate it is a possession of mine; so it's separate from the whole me, just a part of me."

Then with a seemingly adversarial but actually a complimentary trump, Quigley rejoined, "what about your ego, are you separate from that as well?"

The two sipped in silence, as their eyes searched back and forth for deliverance from what Quigley referred to as the ferment of Chardonnay talk. Yet, their minds stiffened, as did their postures as it came to them. In a spark of enlightenment, they started talking simultaneously, not hearing but really understanding each other. They now knew they were separate from their egos and also their minds. These things, these symbols of self, were just parts of their whole selves.

Kaminski's mouth supercharged now, burst into an alcohol-assisted monolog for which he was known. "I know what the mind is; I know what Borges means. The mind is the talking and thinking-in-words part of our brains. It is only a part of our total selves. No one has fully appreciated that when the word, 'mind' came into human language usage centuries ago, it referred to the acknowledgement of the voice inside the head, the voice that could think, write down thoughts and use the word, 'I'. When that word was created it was the beginning of the first awareness of man's understanding that in addition to his spirit and his soul, there was this thinking thing that was called the 'mind'. Even today we keep using the word 'mind' as if it were separate from the body. We can't get away from Cartesian dualism, from *the ghost in the machine* thinking. But the truth is the mind is part of the brain and only part of our entire being; as the ego is just a part of our mind."

Quigley stroked his anemic goatee. "It isn't going to be hard to explain to my wife that I am really not all in my right mind."

In this theory of the mind, it was established in the last chapter that vertical self-identity deals with the evolved layers of increasingly complex sensing and responding neuron systems of the brain. The layered vertical neuron components have been designated as typical of certain types of evolved animals. We consider four layers are present in which the reptile plays a pivotal and primary role. It has been further pointed out that the vertical integration of each of these increasingly complex layers of the self makes it possible for humans to utilize any one or a combination of the components at any given time. There are occasions when reasoning is not effective in survival and only the savagery of combat is. It is also appreciated that certain senses became more developed for the types of evolved animals that represent these layered components of the human brain. In humans, the senses are vision and hearing while in the old mammals, it is the sense of smell.

Horizontal integration of human self-identity refers to the process of uniting the bilateral halves of each of the vertical increasingly complex component layers of the brain.

A gross anatomical inspection of the brain reveals there are two large hemispheres. Each hemisphere is connected to the other with a bridge of tissue, but there are three other important connections that are not quite visible. The vertical axis of the brain has its North-South poles we consider the top and the bottom of the brain. Within the two vertical halves are the horizontal layers of vertical components lying at right angles to that axis. Each layer has two halves and each layer has a bridge of brain tissue connecting the two halves.

The self is a bilateral entity that reflects this anatomical arrangement. **There are actually two sides of the self.** Human duality separates us from the rest of the animal world as much as our ability to communicate with visual and auditory symbols does. (The philosophic and religious authorities of the past projected the internal brain predicament onto the external forces of good and evil.) Gooch serves us well in the understanding of human duality as he reviews the long history of the human suspicion that there are two of us in one body. However, it was Robert L. Stevenson in his novel, *The Strange Case of Dr Jekyll and Mr. Hyde*, who intuitively appreciated the duality was not induced by external evil but an internal mental process.

Each side of the conscious self consists of one half of four vertically integrated layers of increasing complexity and the two sides of these layers each utilize the five senses. We have previously described these layers as (1) reptilian, (2) paleo-mammalian, (3) neo-mammalian, and (4) hominid-human. The layers of the two halves together have been thought of as "different mentalities" by MacLean, but it's worth repeating that in his model there were only three layers, reptilian, paleo-mammalian, and neo-mammalian. Unlike MacLean's prototype, this model has four layers that can also be appreciated as different older brains, each having their two sides joined together. Not resembling any simple geometric figure, the brain looks more like a double head of cauliflower with one stalk. There are connections of the two heads as well as to certain structures below them. These horizontal connections are necessary so that information from one source, sound, for example, coming into one ear is bilaterally integrated into both sides of the brain with the exception of the most complex layers that appreciate sound symbols only on one side and vision symbols on the other.

The first horizontal integrating connection from below upwards is called (1) **the hippocampal commissure.** It joins the bilateral halves of the ancient reptilian layer of the human brain. We remember that the reptilian layer is commonly thought to be part of the limbic system of the brain, but in this theory it is considered to be separate and it consists of two cortical-nuclear elements known as the paired amygdalae and the paired hippocampi which are the prime movers of reptilian behavior in man. The connecting bridge of the next more complex and higher layer is called (2) **the posterior and anterior commissures.** These structures join the two halves of the paleo-mammalian layer of the brain. In man, we consider the two sides of the cingulate cortex to be representative. The next higher and evolved horizontal connection is called (3 and 4) the **corpus callosum**. Its lower connections join the two sides of the more evolved (primate) anthropoid brain and its higher connections join the human-hominid brain. Both cortical structures joined by the corpus callosum are known as the neopallium. See figure (7-1)

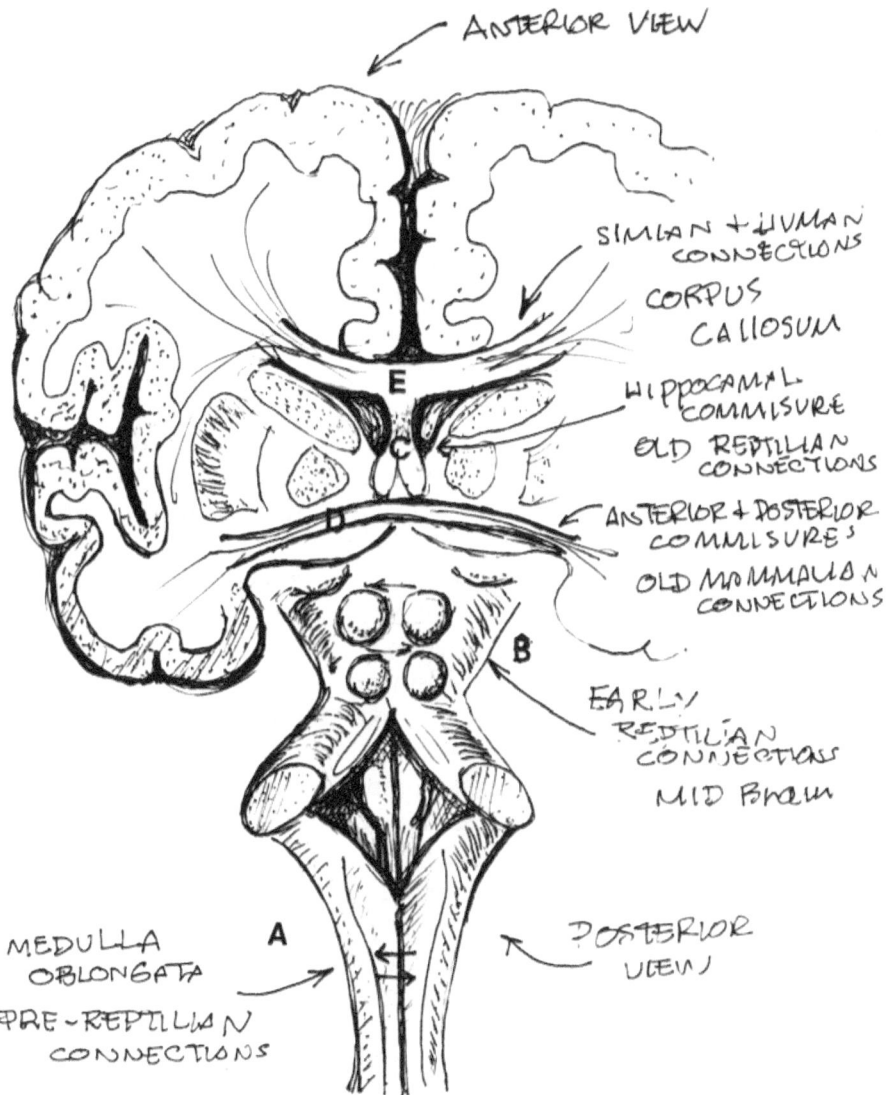

Figure (7-1) A schematic of the horizontal neuronal structures that unite the fundamental paired components of self-identity. Inter-nuclear connections within the medulla oblongata; pre-reptilian type at A. Inter-nuclear connections within the mid brain; early reptilian type at B. Inter-nuclear connections between the cortices of the later land-evolved reptiles, (1) the *hippocampal commissure* at C. Inter-cortical connections of the old mammal brain, (2) *the anterior and posterior commissures* at D. The inter-cortical connections between the cortices of the neo-mammalian brain (anthropoids) as well as the human and hominid cortices, (3 and 4) *the corpus callosum* at E.

Horizontal integration of the nervous system has had a long evolution and to understand the process in humans, it is necessary to take a moment to understand how groups of neurons evolved to be integrated horizontally. After the evolution of the neuron and synaptic processing of sensory information into survival behavior for the organism, an epochal advancement in the nervous system took place with the evolution of **bilateral symmetry**. It started with small organisms like worms that took on sides, a front end and a hind end to their bodies. At the front were the early sensory organs that sensed prey, avoided predators and found mates. The front end had more neurons to accommodate the function of the sensory organs there. When bilateral brain symmetry hit the streets, it became evident with the appearance of sensory organs that came in pairs, one for each side of the animal. One front end **ganglion** *(definition: a collection of nerve cells that serves as a center of nervous influence)* took care of the sense organ on one side of the organism and the other ganglion took care of the opposite side. Eventually the ganglions became connected to make a very primitive brain typical of arthropods. See figure (7-2).

When one looks at a land crab running sideways across a Caribbean beach, if you look close enough when he stops, he has some interesting antennae coming out of the top of his head. You will notice that there is one on each side of his head. They are like their ocean-bound ancestors who as navigators in the sea of predators, mates and prey had bilateral sensors. Animals without bilateral symmetry to their tiny brains had a very inefficient process of sensing prey, avoiding predators and finding mates. It was a hit or miss circumstance in which their principal sense organ acted like one bearing on a compass to locate the object of interest. Where on that bearing line was the object? It could take days of valuable time to chase down the object. With two sense organs, the problem was greatly simplified. Where the two bearing lines of the compass intersected, there lay the object of prey, mating or predatory escape. For example, the segmented worm with its two sided brain and the two sense organs associated with it maneuvers around after an object. First one side sense organ gets a fix and in a millisecond of movement, the other side sense organ gets a fix. Where they intersect lies the object.

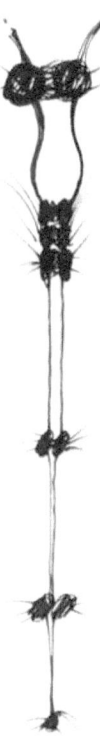

Figure (7-2) A schematic of the bilateral paired ganglionic nervous system of an arthropod, an animal in evolution before those with backbones, the vertebrates. The nervous system is united at its sensing front end by a pool of neurons assembled for sensory input and eventual output to the body.

The sense organs of vision best describe this situation. In primitive animals with bilateral symmetrical brains, that is with two sides, one side is on its own sizing up the environment without any respect to the other side that is sizing up its side of the environment. When one side sees an object stimulus in its side of the environment, something very interesting happens, the animal moves to orient its long axis toward the object of interest so that triangulation can take place. This simple maneuver requires that there is a course change brought about by the muscular components of each side. On the side that first picked up stimulus, more activity takes place and on the other, less activity occurs. The helmsman shifts the power to the side necessary to change direction to face the object. The chameleon aptly demonstrates this neurological mechanism because it has extraordinary excursion and rapidity of movement of its eyes that act independently of one another wherein one can be looking ahead and the other can be looking behind. However, when an insect is seen by one eye, the eyes suddenly become coordinated in extreme convergence so that both are brought to bear upon the prey. This new symmetrical interaction that consists of two separate sensory motor circuits likely takes place by rapid alternation of action of one side to the other. When one side is "on", the other is switched "off" back and forth until an object of survival interest comes into view.

It is speculated that animals with visual sense organs on the far sides of their heads have this arrangement. There is no double vision or confusion where objects are in space because of this alternating switching of the panorama of the visual environment. These wall-eyed creatures can line things up when ready for attack by a switching compass-like action we refer to as "parallax". We can watch chickens turning their heads from side to side to get this form of alignment to peck at a piece of grain.

Animals whose eyes are located on the frontal planes of their heads acquired a greater coordination of the two images that in humans is called **stereopsis**. This new coordinating system provides for some sensory neurons to go to both sides of the symmetrical brains of animals. Stereopsis is what airline pilots need to judge depth perception well enough to land an aircraft safely. It is what an ophthalmologist attempts to get back when an infant is born with a crossed eye that can cause double vision. Very often the doctor is happy when the patient achieves the old way of using two eyes that can't acquire ultimate depth perception or stereopsis. The patient must compensate with what is called **alternation**, or switching back and forth from one eye to the other like long ago ancestors.

The first symmetrical brains of creatures had a very simple neuro-mechanism to utilize both sides of their sensory organs and to activate both sides of the neurons that controlled movement. With the ever increasing complexity of brains and the need for integration of all the senses into a unified motor act, that neuro-mechanism also had to become more complex. The complexity involved coordinating more than one sensory system appropriate in a watery environment to join together in a specific survival motor action. The sense organs of which water olfaction or the chemical sense was most important, worked from side to side by means of a simple mechanism switching back and forth, directing the organism to the object of its interest. This mechanism that united the two sides of early creatures' simple brains of ganglions and small lobes could not manage vertebrate activities after they got curious about living on terra firma. Then, we see coordination of the sensory systems of survival take on a drastic new form because the need to survive in both an aqueous and dry land environment required different means to do so. For those intrepid creatures, it was no longer wise to keep the olfactory system called the chemical sense, to manage survival needs on land. The sense organs had to adapt. Air olfaction took it up a notch and evolved. Vibration stripes along the side of the body didn't work in air. (Remember the cochlear auditory nerve first appeared in amphibians.) Vibration recognition had to change. It required the ability to recognize sound vibrations in air. Vision got in on the act because light energy is more able to stimulate eyes in air than water. There were no good swimming goggles then; eyes were subordinate to water olfaction until animals came ashore. The simple coordinating systems of the water confined animals now were faced with duty on land. About this time, life on land resulted in a new development of the brain first identified in amphibians and reptiles as a "cortical" arrangement of nerve cells. A cortex had a much greater ability to handle more complex functions on land. Evolution was faced with a need for animals to handle the mixed environments. It was not a process as abrupt as Balboa planting his flag or MacArthur wading ashore. It was likely an extended epoch in which the two environments had to be managed over millions of years. The switching mechanism had to evolve further now because two layers of brain sensory tissue were present, one for water, the ganglion, and a new one called a cortex, for land.

This theory proposes that for reptiles and amphibians living in both environments, the simple switching sensory-motor functions of each side of their brains evolved to become the precursors of structures in humans known as **the bilateral hippocampi and the basal ganglia or nuclei.** The hippocampi coordinate the sensory input and the latter coordinate the motor output. Currently it is appreciated that these reptilian structures called the hippocampi and the basal ganglia are necessary to integrate several kinds of sensory information that results in a specific motor behavior. The hippocampi are also appreciated as vital to the functions of memory, especially short term memory. When memory fails in certain diseases, the hippocampal regions are often to blame. In those cases, it is speculated that the hippocampi and the basal ganglia lose their functions of collecting or integrating sensory information from the different sensory cortices and executing a short term motor act related to that sensory integration. Presently in our understanding of hippocampal functions, there is some consideration that they not only bring about memory, but they may also inhibit it because of the basic inhibitory functions of neurons. In this light, it is entirely feasible to understand the observations of Freud who had no knowledge of inhibitory neuronal action, but noted in his patients a peculiar blocking of certain words and names during sensitive interviews.

With this evolutionary background regarding integration of the senses by the hippocampi, we can more readily understand the two sides of the self are integrated as well, so that we think we are just one self. Rightly so, but there are still two symmetrical appearing, vertically aligned hierarchies of brain layers that must be coordinated to keep the organism with a singleness of purpose to match what seems to be a single body. But is human behavior always characterized by a singleness of purpose? The answer is decidedly no. Human nature is fraught with behavior that is very often at cross purposes. One side says one thing while the other does something entirely different. It will come to pass that the asymmetry of the newest cerebral hemispheres are often not in sync and we watch humans doing the most stupid things that even involve criminality.

Looking at Figure (7-3) will help the reader understand the functions of the hippocampi in humans from an evolutionary and anatomical point of view. Switching from one side of the brain to the other in primitive organisms simply told the animal what the senses on each side were picking up in the two sided environment. Both sides of their brains were essentially the same. Primitive animal awareness and responses were simple, (the four "f"s). Very often one sensory organ was more developed than the others. For reptiles, the olfactory sensory system was more developed even before it had a cortex. The new cortex was on each side of the brain and was of equal complexity and capability. In figure (7-3), the transitional water-land reptiles at A, show that bilateral symmetry of the cortical and ganglion levels with their connections that provided the switching back and forth mechanism. At level B, there is diagrammed the more evolved cortex for the major senses along with the most complex, the sense of air olfaction that is typical of old mammals. At level C, the more evolved cortices for the major senses show an additional larger cortical layer for primates that includes a greater complexity for visual and auditory functions. At level D, the human cortical level of the sensory organs, it can be seen that on the right, the visual cortex is more developed and on the left, the auditory cortex is more developed.

All of these cortical elements are shown to have two sides and all levels utilize the switching mechanism, the hippocampi, to take advantage of information coming from one side to the other. The lower levels reveal symmetry of the sides, that is, both sides are the same, except at the human level, there is asymmetry. The sides are different with respect to the most evolved cortex, but regardless of that, those differences are fused as if they were manifestations of one kind of sensation. It appears that the switching, integrating mechanism continues to perform between asymmetrical sides just as easily as it does from symmetrical sides. In so doing, the left side of the brain dominated by auditory functions gets information from the other side dominated by visual functions. By the same arrangement, information from the right gets information from the left. This interaction takes place because of the interconnecting neurons that go back and forth across the large bridge of tissue called the corpus callosum. The two sides of the self subjectively appear as one, but the dominating, controlling auditory half that provides humans with an inner voice and a mind that can think in words attempts to be in control of the other side which has been called the "dark side" of the self, the animus or the anima, the non-dominant, neglected or competitive hemisphere.

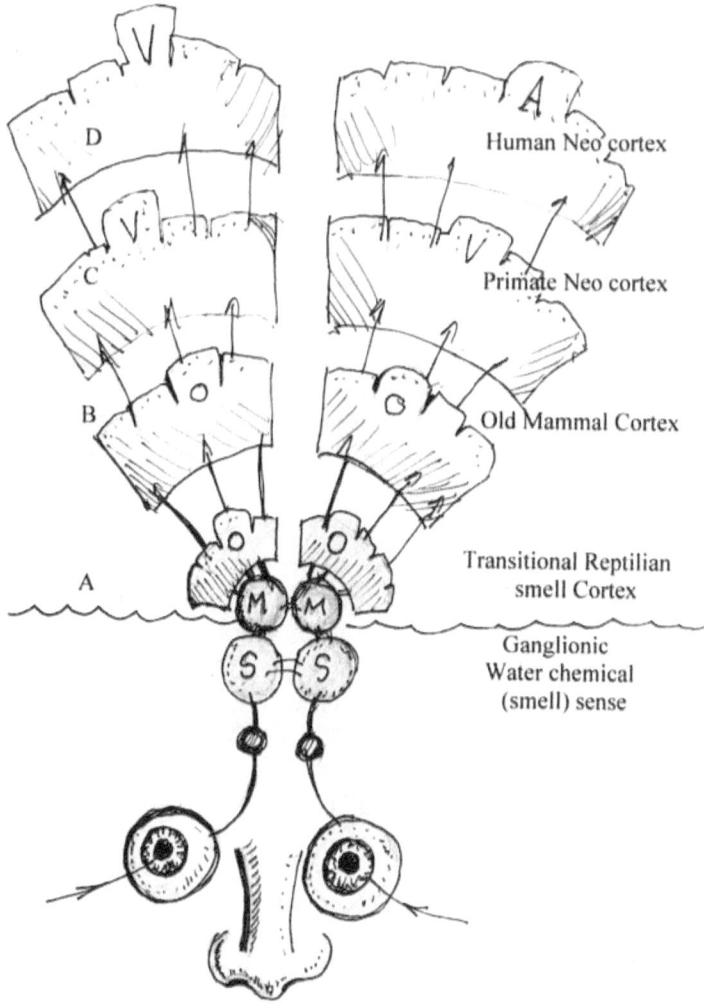

Figure (7-3) The functions of the hippocampi in humans from an evolutionary and anatomical point of view.

Clinical studies from neuropathology reveal the different functions of each side of the brain, but our past thinking has been confined to dominance of one hemisphere with respect to motor control of having right side and hand dominance and having just one side that controls auditory communication. No real attention has focused on the intellectual or personality dominance until recent split-brain studies. However, the modern research of split-brain individuals, as reviewed by Springer and Deutsch also has not understood that the individual sense of self is not always determined by the so-called dominant left hemisphere. Rather it is a state of dynamic flux between the dominant and non-dominant sides of the self. We consider the left hemisphere of the brain as our conscious, rational self, the thinking and speaking dominant self; it takes credit for who we think we are; it takes credit for human self identity. It however fails to appreciate that the other hemisphere causes ongoing changes in the sound of words, the choice of words and the behavior that originates from that side. The silent, unconscious, emotional side of our self is having its say, but in a subtle manner not perceived by the average person in his "right mind".

Springer and Deutsch elaborate on the research with split-brain individuals who are unable to receive any communication from one side of the brain to the other because of a severed corpus callosum. These individuals perform as if they were two separate selves in one body. These subjects, along with other individuals who have suffered strokes to one side of the brain, have provided researchers with information regarding the asymmetrical functions of the highest neocortical levels in man and allowed them to apply this information to "normal" individuals. As Springer and Deutsch point out, in the normal human with a corpus callosum intact, there is often a deceitful explanation of the behavior of the silent-visual-emotional half of the self by the dominant auditory "mind" half. Split brain research explains that humans are unaware of their non-dominant sides, make excuses, cover up or rationalize their behaviors that have their origins in the right hemisphere. An awareness of the right hemisphere's influence allows us to understand what people mean when they have a "gut feeling" about a decision to be made, when the logic of the circumstance is overridden by an emotional feeling.

The influence of the right hemisphere upon the left is further validated in the seminal work of Laing, who noted immature or poorly integrated patients, some normal variants and others including psychopaths and schizophrenics are being controlled by their monkey-child-emotional brain half. Laing's work points out that these individuals unknowingly pretend to be what they say they are and actually use language deceitfully. To some extent, this is a normal set of circumstances for modern humans. In the civilizing process of children with their unbridled sense of emotional omnipotence, it is necessary to inhibit that early behavior. In the process, there appears a normal kind of duality in which for the purpose of social integration and success, child behavior consisting of animal emotions is to be controlled. Yet, that early sense of self remains tucked away in the right hemisphere. If the early development of the emotional-visual child does not provide for a healthy expression of its early characteristics, then the individual does not mature to real adulthood as a "mind" of his left hemisphere. He remains hidden with the pathology of his early years. In the range of "normal", then, we see the multiplicity of behaviors that often present an unconscious deceit in which a "nice" sociability is presented externally to the social world on one hand, but what takes place behind the closed doors of private life is another matter. John or Jane may be wonderful at the bridge table, the athletic club or on the job, but they are hell on wheels at home with their mates because of the way they were reared. If that childhood was really pathological, we appreciate as Laing did, that the right hemisphere plays out its script in the form of child molester, serial rapist, and on and on. Both those who are considered normal or abnormal in our culture use the cover-up of language to deny their asocial behavior and both, for the most part, are unaware of the brain's function in this regard. When language fails, however, the peculiar use of "word salad" by schizophrenics demonstrates the disruption of the left hemisphere by the right.

Gardiner, in his book, *The Shattered Mind*, provides clinical support that the hemispheres compete for control of the brain. The skill in balancing a dowel in one hand is enhanced when one is simultaneously speaking if the dowel is in the left hand, while performance is impaired when one is speaking if the dowel is in the right hand. He explains that speaking and balancing are competing activities when the same side of the brain is doing both acts and they interfere with one another and yet, they promote and facilitate one another when opposite sides of the brain are used simultaneously. With respect to the history of our thinking about right or left cerebral dominance, in the early 1970's, two psychoanalysts, Bandler and Grinder brought to our attention that Milton H. Erickson, M.D., the world's most esteemed Freudian psychoanalyst, using hypnotic techniques in his treatment of the mentally ill, applied the terms "conscious and unconscious" to describe how he was able to induce a trance or state of hypnosis from the conscious mind state to the unconscious mind state. Grinder and Bandler transposed Erickson's terms to "left hemisphere" for the conscious state and "right hemisphere" for the unconscious state of their patients. The new terms laid the groundwork for Wilson's previously quoted statement that the "right hemisphere is the gateway to the unconscious". Most consider that the self is hardly two parts except for a now unpleasant reminder of the Freudian past of a conscious self and an unconscious self.

Clinical studies from split brained patients also reveal that the switching-integrating mechanism evolved further with the advent of asymmetry. In humans, each side of the brain does not have equal access to the emotions going on in lower brain levels. It comes to our attention that the right side of the brain expresses the emotions. Essentially the latest function of the hippocampi is to switch from the auditory mind to the mind of vision along with the emotions of the lower levels of the brain. The hippocampal switching and integrating mechanism also allows a way to access different cortical layers and provides a continuum of behavior that ranges from primitive reptilian behavior to mating and rearing pacific behavior to other highly organized social behaviors. In a metaphoric sense, the hippocampi take the temperature of the environment and integrate actions for dealing with it by consulting each of its bilateral sides. Depending on the temperature of each half, a complex but specific behavior can be activated.

In the newer elements of man's neo-cortices, the **vertical** neuronal reciprocal stimulation and inhibition that are characteristic of all the layers that preceded them, change to become **horizontal** because of the asymmetry of each side. This departure from vertical symmetry that has provided unified animal behavior contrarily has created a chance for conflict between the two asymmetrical sides of the brain in humans. The human mind that creates words can get easily separated from the emotions. These emotions can cause asocial body acts that the word brain attempts to cover up with lies and excuses.

It is important to point out that the first asymmetry of the human brain began with the further evolution of the monkey symmetrical, visually dominated brain. In experiments on monkeys who have been taught a mixed form of visual sign language and auditory language wherein verbal sounds from a human can activate a visual symbol response, one begins to grasp man's evolution to asymmetrical auditory dominance. The experiments suggest that these monkeys are artificially triggered into expressive communication with visual symbols, but they are clearly stimulated by visual body language in the wild. That primate evolution led to early man's ability to communicate with visual hand signs and then drawn symbols. In this way, early humans controlled their clan members and began to inhibit their monkey emotional inclinations. (This form of visual communication-intelligence has gone on to play a significant role in human symbolic intelligence and in the written communication we find characteristic of Asian races.) In human evolution, when auditory language superseded visual silent communication, there was a shift in neo-cortical dominance from right to left. In evolutionary time, we have suggested it didn't take long.

Humans are in a transit of evolution in which there is a struggle to rid behavior from dominance of one side of the brain over the other. Evolution of mankind is in the lethal grip of the brain's progress in this regard because symbolic brain functions, both right and left, produce technology to continue old reptilian eruptions in human behavior. From an individual perspective, the ontogeny of the issue, in addition to the phylogenetic one of survival of the human species, we see the writhing of cerebral dominance in excessive inhibition of the emotional and visual side of humans' right hemispheres in the form of robotic oppression, timidity, depression and other mental dysfunctions. On the other hand, in the absence of inhibition by the left auditory-verbal hemisphere, we witness the fleshing out of hedonistic and sadistic behavior of the past. Can evolution that is attempting to bring equilibrium between the two asymmetrical sides of the brain make it in time before the brain destroys the species? In the present state of brain evolution, the competitive and cooperative interactions have to do with the auditory left symbolic neo-cortex acting in a process of civilizing the older right neo-cortex of monkeys and their emotions by the voice and acts of civil reason. It provides a mind that attempts to control the animal acts of emotion, to regulate them for survival among great numbers of humans who take a long time to mature, proliferate rapidly and are prone to the many problems of not accurately recapitulating the steps of their evolution.

The hippocampal switching-integrating mechanism within the reptilian core of the human brain provides a state of the union between the two different parts of our intellectual and emotional natures. It assesses how things are going on each side of the brain. If the left auditory symbolic cortex is poorly developed because of a lack of entraining from others, the lower emotional behaviors and body acts are used as survival techniques although they may be neither socially acceptable nor effective. Entraining in humans is a long, delicate process, in which the emotional side of the brain can't be rigidly inhibited as we just mentioned, because the emotional side needs an appropriate expression in order to be healthy and in equilibrium with its other half. We need to appreciate that the great purpose of the right cortex, in addition to providing a different kind of higher intelligence, is to activate emotional body behavior, while the effect of the left cortex is to inhibit it. The two neo-cortical hemispheres are in equilibrium when each side has a balanced expression. This relationship can be inferred from pathology that results from a stroke in the left neo-cortex. When that occurs, there is a release from inhibition of the right hemisphere and a greater expression of the emotions occurs. A stroke on the opposite side causes a diminished expression of emotions.

The human self, we now see, is not just that part of the brain we have called "the mind" that seems to tell ourselves as well as others who we "think" we are. The self, rather, is the two sides of the brain and the two great mentalities that retain evolved layers of animal self-identity of the distant past. It also includes a core element of those two cerebral hemispheres and that core provides us with our basic human emotional consciousness in the form of fear and anger. It also provides humans the ability to access all of our more developed senses and behaviors.

To appreciate this core self and its integrative-coordinating mechanism which is located in the diencephalon of the forebrain, we must turn specifically to the genius of another past investigator, Wilder Penfield. Through his clinical findings in the late part of the 1900's, we can better understand how the brain works with regard to having a reptilian core self-identity and an integrating mechanism for the many special senses of the self, especially the two senses of vision and of hearing in the higher neo-cortices. Penfield, a neurosurgeon, was one of those early scientists who began the transformation of thinking about the mind and its relationship to the brain.* He drew attention to a consideration previously reviled by many, that the mind had some fleshy brain parts. Penfield was not only a neurosurgeon of world renown, but also a man who was perplexed as to where the mind was in the brain. He had an excellent opportunity to study what happened to the brain when certain parts were missing due to epilepsy. During operations attempting to cure that disease, he came upon the most significant data concerning where the nuclear core of the self and an integrating mechanism of the senses were located. Penfield's work on the epileptic disease of petit mal fleshed out a profound insight. "In this disease there are attacks of *automatism*. A patient becomes suddenly unconscious, but since another mechanism in the brain continues to function, he changes into an automaton. He may wander about confused and aimless. He may continue to carry out whatever purpose his mind was in the act of handing on to his automatic sensory-motor mechanism. He can follow a stereotyped, habitual pattern of behavior for a short time. In every case, he will not be able to make decisions and he makes no record of what has happened, he cannot remember what had happened to him during an attack. In these attacks he may become completely unreasonable and uncontrollable and even

---

* The Frenchman, Lamettrie, planted the seed of philosophical materialism that began the transformation of the mind as a separate psychology to a manifestation of neuro-biology.

dangerous." In his work, Penfield demonstrated that the part of the brain affected by petit mal epilepsy occurs from injury not specifically in the higher cortices of the brain but in the lower and older part of the brain.

Epileptic seizures may appear to begin in the prefrontal and temporal lobes and cause petit mal automatism but the actual source of the automatism begins in the diencephalon or higher brain-stem. When out of action from the seizure this older central part of the brain is disconnected from the prefrontal cortex, the decision-making part of the mind. It is separated from all kinds of other cortical functions that include on-going or past events from our varied senses, both long term and short-term memory. In addition to the separation from memory and the decision-making process, the diencephalic mechanism of self-identity is also separated from the thinking auditory symbolic cortex in the left hemisphere and from the right visual association cortex as well. In petit mal, the brain's motor functions "proceed along temporarily having been directed prior to the attack." A body is there doing things and the motor cortex of the brain that moves muscles to do those things is there for a short time, but there is no real person, no *self*, only a mindless robot. From these observations, Penfield concluded that there is a site of central gray matter in the higher brain-stem that is affected by petit mal which causes a zombie-like state of consciousness. This area is located at the level of the thalamus and the basal ganglia in the human diencephalon. (See figure (7-4.) It corresponds to the "R-complex" of MacLean and to a "nucleus of the self" as defined by other investigators. It is this location that accounts for the unique neurological condition called decerebration and decortication in which a patient is unconscious and exhibits spastic contraction of his extremities.

Penfield believed that the part of the mind he called the "highest brain mechanism" was anatomically located in the ancient vertebrate part of the forebrain called the diencephalon. If the mind had a brain mechanism, it is likely Penfield initially posited that the mind was a neuronal brain structure. In his popular expose, *The Mystery of the Mind*, he revealed his absorption with his dilemma. Initially he set out to prove the mind was part of the brain, but over time, he returned to a dualistic appreciation of the mind and the brain as separate.

Penfield's highest brain mechanism and the primitive cortex of the amygdalae are at the site of reptilian self-identity neurons that give rise to the consciousness of fear and anger; it is the portion of the old brain of mammals from which MacLean draws his conclusions about reptilian behavior that provides humans with their basic survival instincts. It also contains the mechanism for multiple sensory integration for action derived from the hippocampi and the automatic motor behavior initiated by the hippocampi.

Penfield identified this central nuclear core of self-identity in a patient whose neurological problem was the opposite of that found in petit mal. In this fascinating case, the patient presented with an injury in which the central core of the brain remained intact, but was disconnected from the cortical components of the brain by an extensive hemorrhage. Penfield could see by observing the eyes of his patient that he was still alive, primitively conscious. Yet he had no other observable functions of the mind. Penfield went on to explain that this nuclear core of consciousness interacted with all the cortical components of the brain through an automatic sensory-motor mechanism adjacent to the core self-identity neurons in the diencephalon. Today we appreciate the automatic sensory motor mechanism and the highest brain mechanism he described are the symmetrically, evolved reptilian core neurons of the self in the diencephalon. That core includes the amygdalae, the hippocampi and the basal nuclei. See figure (7-5).

For many years, abnormalities of the basal nuclei were considered by neurologists to be simply strange disorders of motion known as reduced (hypokinetic) or increased (hyperkinetic) disturbances. Some of these abnormalities in motion are known as ballismus, choreiform movements, athetoid movements, akinesia and bradykinesia. Diseases such as Huntington's chorea, Parkinson disease and Sydenham chorea provided neurological evidence of the basal nuclei's function.

Recent appreciation of the function of the basal nuclei shows us that these areas are concerned with the "automatic motor mechanism" Penfield described in petit mal epilepsy. Huntington's disease, Alzheimer's disease and Parkinson's disease demonstrate the many associated defects, such as memory loss, planning movements, psychiatric disorders and affective disorders, associated with reptilian mechanisms of behavior.

Researchers, in addition to Penfield, have demonstrated that if this switching area and its automatic action system are isolated and removed from brain function in many vertebrates including humans, intentional actions including perception and learning are lost. It is the deeply located central old brain of reptiles and an evolved part of its cortex, the hippocampi and basal nuclei that provide final multi-sensory integration and orientation in time and space with reciprocal connections to all the sensory and motor cortices of both the old and new brain of the human.

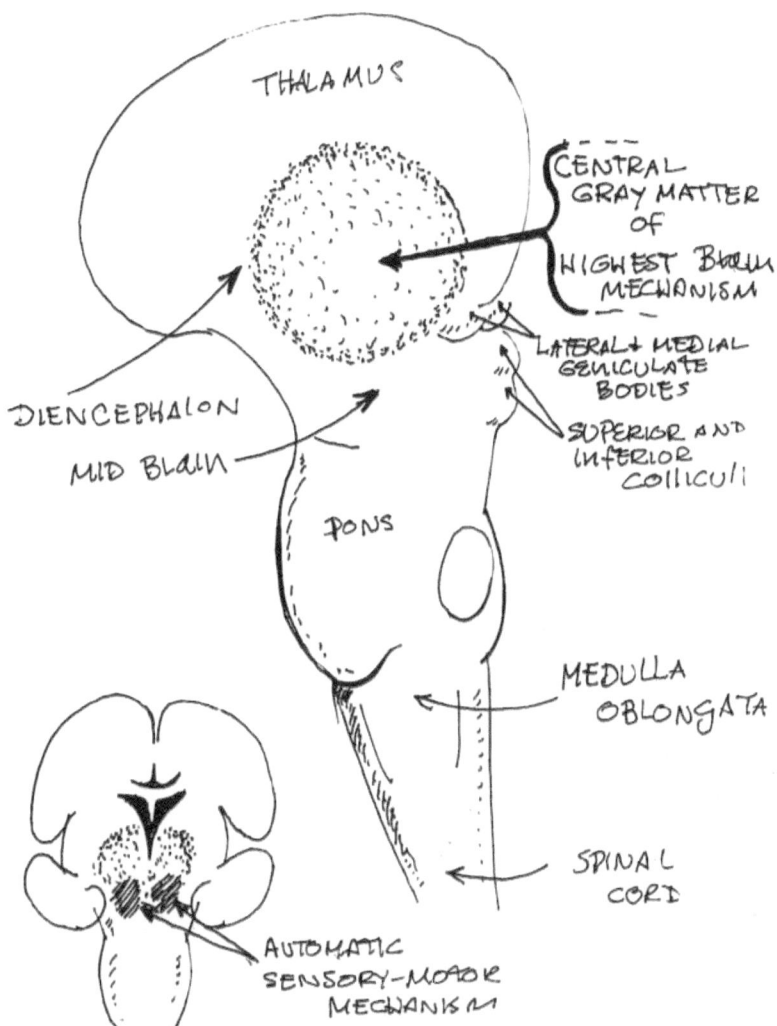

Figure (7-4) From Penfield's illustration of the location of the core element of the mind.

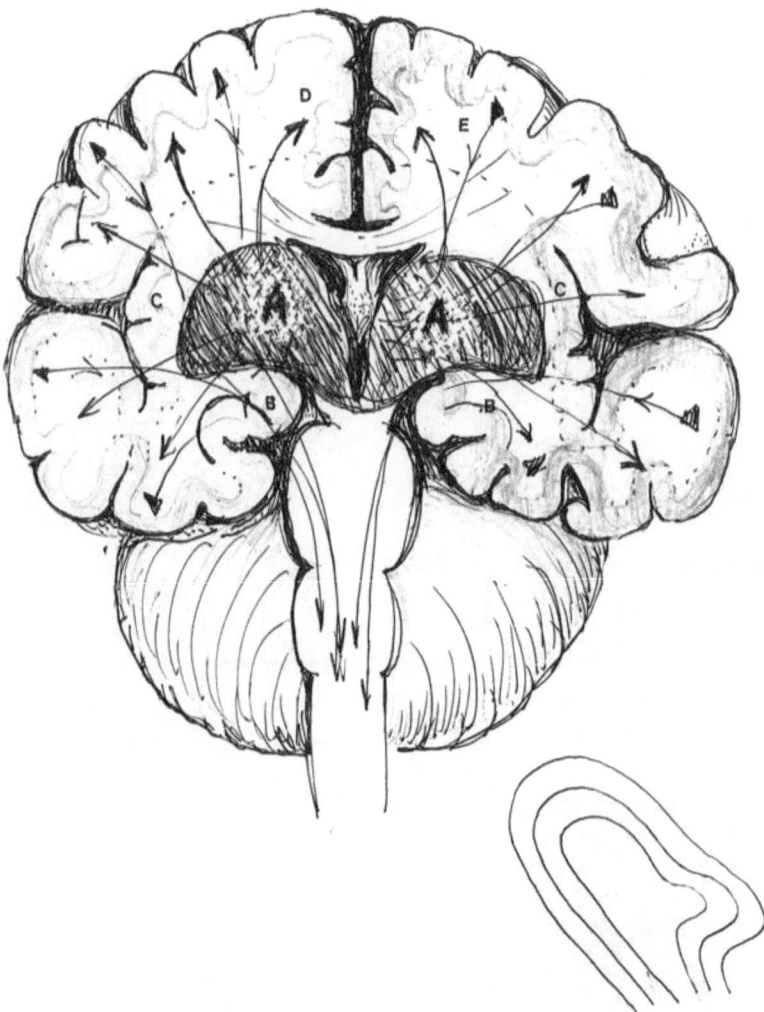

Figure (7-5) Penfield's highest brain mechanism (A), a primary switching station within the diencephalon with connections to the archicortical structures of the amygdalae and hippocampi of reptilian origin at (B), to the paleocortical structures of paleo-mammalian origin at (C), and to the intellectualcortical structures of neomammalian and human origin at (D) and (E).

Let's examine how vertical and horizontal integration work in an old mammal, the lion. His cortical, sensory-motor functions are wired for easy to see behaviors of reproducing, preying or being preyed upon. Take being preyed upon as an example. First, the animal smells a tiny odorant; he is downwind to the predator. His olfactory sensory cortex is (microscopically) activated. The initial contact proceeds to activate neurons in his pre-reptilian mid-brain where a general alarm is sounded; the alarm clock goes off for the first time. Then the stimulus activates the archipallium, initially on the side the smell is coming from and then on the other. In the hippocampi, there are no other signals arriving from the senses of hearing or vision on either side of the brain. The process essentially is a one sensory event that effects the animal's behavior. The appropriate motor response for this small amount of input results in a small amount of automatic output. The animal is aroused only; he sits up and listens and looks. Then, as the predator comes within hearing range and the smell of the predator continues to become more intense, the hippocampi receive a stronger signal. This results in a two sensory process that summates to bring about even more watchful behavior; the animal gets up and assumes a fight or flight posture. Finally, as the predator comes even closer so that it can be seen as well as heard and smelled even more intensely, the lion snaps into fight or flight motor behavior. Essentially, the three senses work together to reach the threshold of synaptic motor activity for full survival against a predator. The hippocampal population of neurons acts within its synapses by means of positive or negative feedback from each sensory system. At times the hippocampi provide a summation or positive feedback for action, at other times a steady state of action, and at still others negative feedback to create inaction.

HUMAN ASYMMETRY

This theory of the self, the asymmetrical division of neo-cortical hemispheric functions is not limited to the well-known and accepted differences between the two. The currently defined differences are the parietal association area of the right hemisphere that deals with space relationships and selective attention functions and the left inferior frontal and superior temporal lobe areas that deal with auditory symbolic language. Rather, as split brain and other studies confirm, there is a host of intellectual functions of the two halves of the brain that exceed simple auditory language on the one hand, and the simple spatial relationships on the other. *This understanding of the functions of each neo-cortical hemisphere proposes that the asymmetry includes almost the entire neo-*

cortex. It includes the prefrontal lobe and the temporal lobe, the occipital lobe as well as the accepted parietal area.

We have no difficulty in appreciating the asymmetry of motor function that further defines this global hemispheric difference, but I don't believe that neuroscience fully appreciates that one half of the human brain's intellectual function is based principally on vision and the other half on sound. Nor is it fully appreciated that there is a long evolution of visual communication of symbols that can also be considered language. We recall, for example, there is the omission of visual symbolic evolution in Jaynes' theory of the origin of consciousness in the bicameral brain because he mistakenly concludes human consciousness began with the evolution of auditory symbolic communication.

It has been forgotten or ignored that visual communicative intelligence all began before the evolution of auditory symbolic communication. There is the Rosetta stone to prove it and there are remnants in this modern world of the obligations of behavior dictated by astrology and horoscopes. It is postulated that in addition to the unimodal neo-cortex of the left hemisphere that relates to the intelligence of auditory symbolic language and the unimodal neo-cortex of the right hemisphere that relates to visual intelligence, what is considered multimodal in the frontal lobes is an integration of the two forms of intelligence. In the normal brain, the two forms of intelligence are integrated, joined by the interaction of neurons by means of the corpus callosum. The data regarding their individual functions are not so much absent but not identified in the respect to the sensory systems from which these functions evolved. The data relate to the different forms of agnosia and apraxia, prosody, emotional dampening or exaggeration and body awareness and space awareness. Rethinking in terms of visual function or auditory function helps us appreciate that the mind with its verbal language must unite with the body and its actions in space, the older emotions and the visual intelligence that it does not possess. The left brain of our mind does not appreciate that the so-called non-dominant right hemisphere is a vital part of our self-identity, personality and our survival.

Of great importance is the present thinking about an undifferentiated visual-auditory function of the prefrontal cortex that has to do with the most keen and sophisticated form of human intelligence. The frontal lobes provide humans with the ability to look ahead, plan for the future, to see themselves clearly as not just body-minds, not just victims of others actions, not as objects of blame in the social process. The lobes also allow humans the ability to "see" themselves in others, not in an unconscious process of projection of negative aspects that really are their own, but in a form of empathy. These are the aspects of what the right visual frontal lobe brings to the table, while it is the ultimate verbal reasoning and decision making of the left auditory frontal lobe that come about with the assistance of visual input from the right.

There is a difference in the judgments and decisions that have been learned by rote of what was put in the heads of those who repeat words and remember words expertly and those decisions that involve seeing ahead and being able to adapt to seeing what's coming down the road of day to day survival. With an understanding of such a division of prefrontal functions as well as the other parts of the two hemispheres, we can explain why the frontal lobes are so important to our ability to think both in words and pictures. It provides us with an explanation as to why some thinking is restricted to linear reasoning and to grammatically correct, narrative thinking, while other thinking has the ability to be picturesque and metaphoric; why one is legal jargon and another is the bountiful imaginative use of words as exemplified by the works of the novelist Lawrence Durrell.

We can further appreciate that visual memories are stored for retrieval in the temporal lobe on the right, while verbal memories are stored for retrieval in the temporal lobe on the left. It tells us that Einstein was a theoretical thinker who spent most of his life not being practical, but deep in his mind seeing the relationships of things others could not see. He was out of the box of the dominating left hemisphere and his entire character wanted freedom from the rigid thinking of what the left hemisphere said was not to be violated. He could get lost walking home because he was up there in his frontal lobes jiggling symbols that had never been united in a symbolic pattern. He was "dancing" back and forth across his corpus callosum seeing and talking with a freedom that rigid left brained thinkers of the past (such as the papal authority) would not have allowed.

EVIDENCE OF HORIZONTAL AND VERTICAL INTEGRATION OF SELF

There is information from the clinical observation of patients that appears to verify the neural substrate of a core of the self with its two halves that are vertically and horizontally integrated. These observations were made while patients were being interviewed by a psychologist. One human, the patient, was interacting with another human, the interviewer. The two individuals were seated and interacting with their two most complex sensory systems of sound and sight. They were looking at each other and talking to each other. The interviewer says: "Now, you have been on this committee for two months. I can't believe that you have not accomplished the goals that we asked you to accomplish. Just what have you been doing for those two months?" The gaze and body position of the interviewer are directly confrontational, a bit angry as judged by the furrowed brow while he says these words. They are said in a no-nonsense style that means business. While these words are being spoken, the patient is looking directly at the interviewer and his eyes are noted to search back and forth at the interviewer, just like the alternating switching back and forth of those primitive land crabs. Some observers have called this a process of *sensory up time*. This fraction of the interchange for the patient is one in which his two involved senses are "receiving" very much like the process that occurs with VHF radio transmission that involves just the auditory sense not the visual and the auditory senses combined. Like the radio transmission, one cannot "send" and "receive" simultaneously when engaged in the process of transmitting with the visual and auditory sensory systems of the brain. During sensory up time, auditory symbolic information and visual body language information are being sensed. The information goes into the brain and the auditory information ends up in the left neo-cortex that can appreciate language symbols and also in the right and left older sound cortex that can appreciate how they are spoken. The visual information goes to the right association neo-cortex that can appreciate visual body language especially facial expressions. The switching of the patient's eyes reveals his nervous system is going back and forth, switching from the auditory sensory system to the visual system so that he can fully appreciate not only the words, but how they are spoken and how the interviewer appears while he is saying them. That appreciation requires a previous imprinting or learning we call memory.

The interviewer expects an answer in word symbols from the patient. To arrange or create an answer, the patient now must access the visual and auditory memories to give a fully comprehensive, intelligent answer. This process is no different than using the VHF radio in which the operator switches off the reception and creates a return message to the caller. This fraction of the interaction has been called *sensory down time*. It is observable by the action of the patient's eyes that now change from a switching back and forth saccadic movement to a diagonal-vertical up and down movement. During the next TV interview, watch how constant these eye movements actually are. Sensory down time occurs when the diencephalic switching mechanism of the old reptile part of the human brain is activated to retrieve and integrate what was said, how it was said and how the interviewer appeared while he said it. Essentially the information from both systems becomes integrated after being assimilated. The digestion, so to speak, is an integration of the two sensory modes of information that involves the pre-frontal lobes whose part in vision and hearing has been explained.

RELATIVE CONSCIOUSNESS

The switching integrating mechanism of the ancient part of the human brain is not only extremely important to an understanding of memory, but what is considered consciousness. Consciousness is defined as "the awareness of one's own existence, sensations, thoughts, surroundings, to be aware". We accept this definition the dictionary provides, but it needs to be further defined here. That awareness of things coming into the mind-brain pretty much covers all the information that comes from all the senses. Any observer might not know how conscious you are if you do not respond to his enquiring verbal stimulus. You, yourself, answer your own internal enquiries in the same way. Of what is each of my complex sensing mechanisms aware, to what degree? This appraisal requires a method of communication that in the conscious state of mind we refer to as auditory language. The psychiatrist-psychologist inquires about your thoughts that are part of your consciousness. Some psychiatrists-psychologists are interested in what we banter around as the "subconscious". The neurologist also is interested in how conscious you are, but to a limited extent that determines if you are conscious of your simple state of being regarding the memory of being aware of time of day, month and year and where you reside. The neurologist is very much interested in how conscious your nervous system is when you can't tell him how conscious you are, when you are unconscious or unable to communicate.

The important consideration is the fact that the nervous system can't be conscious of everything at the same time. As you read this sentence, you can be made aware of the symbolic content of the words and the sentence of which they are an integral part. However, there are many other things at this moment of which you are aware, but your mind must be directed to them to make them fully conscious. Therefore, a great deal of what we are conscious is really subconscious until retrieved by an active mental process utilizing auditory or visual symbolic language. This retrieval is brought about by the old reptile switching-integrating component of the brain. Yet, a great deal of consciousness remains in the background in a state of being subconscious or pre-conscious.

Over time, for instance, the ticking of a clock and even its bell ringing out the hour of the day will cease to be in our active consciousness but will slip into the background or subconscious state. Many old European clocks rang the hour twice because there were so many complaints by individuals who were not conscious of exactly when the bell tower began to ring out the number of the hour. They wanted to hear it a second time when they were fully conscious of the total number of times the bell rang. Being conscious then, once specific sensory neurons have acquired the ability to retain information requires that it be retrieved. It must come from a subconscious state to a conscious state.

"I didn't even hear the clock ticking until you told me to listen to its ticking."

"Yes, I had to draw your attention to it. I had to make you conscious of it. I know that you know the clock is ticking, but you were not aware of it at the moment prior to my telling you to listen."

We recall that in child development, we must learn by auditory language to be conscious of our self-identity with respect to our body parts and all the sensations that our sensory systems provide. "Mommy, my ear hurts," says the child who has learned the words to direct attention to just where the pain of the body is coming. He also eventually learns that he has a mind and emotions as part of his self-identity. It is time for humans to learn that the mind is more than the talking and thinking part of the brain in the left neo-cortex and that it includes many things that we appreciate as subconscious from other parts of the brain. One most important aspect is the silent right hemisphere that represents an evolutionary status of the human species and a sense of self that expresses the emotional child who must pass through this stage to survive in a complex society.

NEUROCEPTIVES AND FEELINGS

Any conscious awareness of the information brought about by the brain's many specialized cortices and their sense organs either in ongoing reality or retrieved from memory in a virtual reality can be thought of as "neuroceptives". They include both horizontal and vertical elements of the self. Therefore, any sensory system can be brought into consciousness and any layer or combinations of those senses can also become conscious.

Neuroceptive is a term derived from the work of Sir Charles Sherrington who received a Nobel prize in 1932 in physiology and medicine. Sherrington is the world famous physiologist who created the word "synapse", a term he introduced to describe the interaction between two neurons. Sherrington also introduced to science three other words involved in human sensory functions: 1. proprioceptive, 2. interoceptive and 3. exteroceptive. These terms refer to sensory receptors that send information to the central nervous system regarding muscle and tendon positions, and organ and skin sensations.

Sherrington's discovery came at a time in history when neuro-physiologists were not aware that certain sensory nerves provided such information to the brain. Ironically, the neuro-physiologists, themselves, were utilizing those sensory parts of the brain in every day life, but were not fully conscious of them. The types of sensory information Sherrington identified can be included in a broad category of sensations that we can bring into consciousness. Neuroceptives are different kinds of sensory information that become part of the mind's conscious awareness when the mind learns to talk about such sensations, when words come to define those sensations that are the special functions of different sensory cortical systems. This communication requires a neuron driven connection between those other cortices and the left auditory symbolic cortex. Neuroscientists have to learn words for the brain's parts and mechanisms, just as children must learn new words for parts of their bodies like the foot and the big toe.

Another neuroceptive mechanism similar to those identified by Sherrington, still remains obscure. It is the old sensory motor self-identity system of children and all those humans and hominids that think in terms of vision and visual symbols and very little in terms of word symbols. That part of human self-identity is the right cerebral neocortex and it is a big part of the mind's total action, but we continue have trouble identifying it in terms of anatomical reality in the form of a neuron system.

The smell of a flower is an example of a primary or real neuroceptive. Without a name to that specific smell, the best humans can describe it would be with a simplistic game of charades that includes holding a specific flower and animating the act of "smelling". If an individual knows the name of a particular flower and can call to conscious memory that flower's particular scent, that individual is fully conscious of the flower's smell. If this process occurs in the absence of the real flower being there in the garden, it can be brought to consciousness by the auditory word cortex of the brain in a process of symbolic memory that can be considered a virtual example of a neuroceptive. "What does Mary Ellen look like?" is a further example of the auditory symbolic left cortex directing the hippocampal mechanism to switch to the visual cortex to retrieve from memory a retained visual neuroceptive. Nausea is another primary neuroceptive that pops into center stage consciousness and it doesn't take much experience of the real event to become connected to the learned word if one is feeling queasy. It may be difficult to believe the ongoing panorama of the visual, external environment is also a specific neuroceptive function of the primary visual cortex, but it's going on like a movie film until a specific visual event in it is brought to attention.

Historically, it is of interest to appreciate that Dr. Sherrington, the physiologist, was no exception to those who believed there was a separation of body-brain from the mind. The brain and its peripheral nerves were part of the body and his discoveries regarding sensations were linked to a neurological manifestation of the brain, not the mind, in his thinking. Neurology was a study of the body-brain, psychology-psychiatry was a study of the mind, and things are still thought of with this division of enquiry. Sherrington did not accentuate nor was he interested in the mind's participation in the appreciation of the memories and specific functions of other parts of the brain, that was the realm of the non-neurological team. So we can guess that he did not know the neuro-mechanism that provides the mind a conscious awareness of his new discoveries. He likely had no interest where the mind was in the brain. Yet, we establish it is specifically the left neocortex described by Broca and Wernicke. Once neurons of auditory language are hooked up with the process of learning with those other brain areas, the mind can talk about them and be fully conscious of them. It now should be clear that when you ask yourself where your right hand is at this moment, if it feels heavy, and if you further ask yourself if you feel hungry or if your nose is cold, you realize that these sensory functions can be brought easily into consciousness by the use of words that direct the hippocampi to switch awareness to a specific sensory system that has the specialized capability of reception.

Words spoken out loud, or under the breath, or thoughts of the internal voice are also a type of neuroceptive of the auditory language sensory-motor cortex, in which the sensory cortex is listening to its motor part. Of great significance are the neuroceptives of the emotional cortices. Current awareness of most humans appreciates that the emotions are something different than the rational mind supposedly doing the talking and thinking. This assumption can be based on the understanding that the emotions are manifestations of older cortical layers of the brain and that we, humans, have put words to their specific type without knowing they are just like the neuroceptives coming from different areas of the brain. When we are conscious of emotional neuroceptives, we refer to them as "feeling" states such as: "I feel good; I feel down; I feel sad; or I am in love." Having a more explicit understanding of human behavior based on anatomical reality is not an attempt to fracture human unity, or its singleness of purpose, but a better way to understand the elements that make up human wholeness.

The specialized neuronal functions of all our senses can be lost, but the self-identity core neurons as Penfield discovered and others have verified, can remain partially conscious without those specialized parts. We need just to look at the aphasic stroke victim, the person that lost certain memory and the patient who is going crazy-losing his mind. There is still a self minus those diseased components.

By way of understanding further how the intact, healthy brain-mind works in this theory of self-identity, we can imagine that all cortical components of the self, both vertical and horizontal are able to listen and talk on a conference call. A call comes to the operator (symbolic auditory cortex).

The caller asks, "How are the body and mind feeling today?" This information is heard by the operator and she connects up with the message center before answering the caller. The center calls each of the self-identity components for their thoughts on the matter.

Somatosensory cortex answers back, "Everything is not quite ok; we are receiving information from the body that there is a pain in the right big toe."

"Thanks," says the message center. Then the center calls every other sensory component regarding their special awareness.

Vision station reports, "I have not seen anything unusual."

Smell station reports, "Things are ok here."

Taste station reports, "We have a dry mouth being identified."

R-complex reports, "That particular caller makes us mad."

Limbic emotional station reports, "Nothing good going on here."

The message center reports all this information to the operator who holds her hand over the phone and talks with her boss, the prefrontal thinking cortex, who decides upon the final reply.

"After reviewing all the responses, I think that this particular caller should not really know how we feel. Tell the caller accordingly, operator."

The operator now knows how the whole human self feels and tells the caller waiting on the line, "I (all of me) feel fine. How are you today?"

While such an analogy is helpful in understanding the horizontal integration of the brain's complete self-identity, it is important not to be deceived, as ancient scientists believed, that the self is just a miniature self inside the deep part of the brain stem. The self is the sum total of its parts, vertical and horizontal. If you damage one of those parts, you take away part of human self-identity. (We recall that confused hominids eventually acquired a brain that could appreciate that what they saw and heard out there in the environment was not actually part of them. They learned through language that objects in nature were separate from their subjective selves.) However, man does not live without environmental stimulation. Vision, for instance, is a physical process going on in a specific brain cortex. Yet, the process involves an environmental energy to create its presence in our awareness.

The vertical integration of the self allows a human to use symbols of auditory language and vision to stimulate and respond at the highest, most complex level of behavior. Yet the system allows the self to regress in a modulated or total fashion to lower (emotional) levels of behavior. In a complimentary way, the horizontal integration of the self allows the human to access all of his sensory mechanisms including sound, vision, smell, taste and touch in this vertical process. The auditory symbolic cortex mediates the control of both systems. With both systems functioning, a normal human is able to make responses with the greatest amount of information from all the senses. In modern urban circumstances, however, the best human judgments are made using the two most evolved senses (auditory and visual) which require the integration of both hemispheres.

By nature of human brain evolution, man is more or less a dualistic creature, because of the divide between the silent, visual-emotional hemisphere and the auditory, symbolic-reasoning hemisphere. When man cannot integrate both hemispheres successfully, he may become a pathologically dualistic human, such as a schizophrenic or a psychopath. The truly pathological dualistic individual is a split, poorly integrated brain in one body. Notorious serial killers, such as Jack the Ripper, Son of Sam, Ted Bundy, and Gary Ridgeway who remain members of a normal society by day, but act out demonic behavior by night are grisly examples. Many of these individuals with pathological dual personalities are conscious of their double nature, but the criminal, who is truly dualistic, is not. The neuro-pathological form of dualistic personality reveals itself in a specific detachment of spoken words (coming from the left hemisphere's symbolic auditory cortex) as well as detachment from the expression of emotions in body language (coming from the right hemisphere). The absence of the left brain's integration with the emotions coming through the right results in a flat tone of voice and visible lack of emotions that identify these pathological individuals.

Even in individuals whom we consider more normal than not, there is this element of duality in which the left side must deal with the right side. If the left side is developed only to the level of dictatorial parenting in its dealing in the world, when the left side cannot appreciate how others feel and deal with them, they respond to any challenge of their limited view of the world with: "No, that's not the way things are, how could you say such a thing?" In these individuals, the right hemisphere is a stunted child who never had the chance to express itself with any freedom from the parental left hemisphere. In others who acquired another form of neurotic/normal behavior, the right side child may have developed some peculiar traits that the left side tries to accommodate by excuses and other defenses, but has no idea of the silent imbedded nature of the so-called neurotic behavior. Jay Haley, an expert in family therapy, described in detail how a young man concerned about his impotency with women identified through therapy that his neurotic behavior was a result of an unconscious childhood disturbance in sexual development. However, contrary to Freudian treatment theory, catharsis is not a simple solution to childhood scarring. Only good parenting can bring about a fully integrated adult self-identity.

In conclusion, the self, an individual's total self identity, consists of all the cortical specialized senses with their accumulated memories, the vertical and horizontal integration of these neuroceptives and the social and intelligent integration of right and left hemispheres. Borges, like so many creative individuals, was aware that new ideas and concepts are not the sole manifestation of the auditory language side of the brain and for the most part, creative thought originates in the images of the silent visual hemisphere. Humans can't readily understand verbal ideas unless they visualize them in a neuroceptive conscious state. Borge's experience tells us that we humans are in a process of acknowledging the self is more than the mind with its voice inside us even though it usually is the captain of the ship.

Chapter 8

Adult Human Ontogeny

How human self-identity acquired from a specific culture can inadvertently cause illness.

Carl Humboldt Fritze was one of the few medical school classmates David Kaminski considered to be a friend. There were many occasions the consideration was in doubt, but overall he felt kinship not animosity toward Fritze. Carl was known in those days of 1953 as a type of legacy to the medical school, because his father had been a physician in a small Canadian border community of the State of Washington. In bygone days before Kaminski got the idea to join the Hippocratic fraternity, it was possible for doctors' sons with few other credentials to be accepted into the medical schools their fathers had attended. The process was often accompanied by the passing of silver from alumni to faculty. The land grant University of Washington was not a private institution that survived on such practices of nepotism. Nonetheless, the new faculty coming mainly from hallowed private institutions was still influenced by the practice. The faculty members were careful, however, to make certain that applicants who were accepted represented every corner of the state where honest taxpayers' dollars supported the school. Some classmates of Kaminski got into medical school after spending only three years in premedical training. These individuals often had unusual academic scores. Kaminski, as well as most other classmates, went through four years of undergraduate school to be accepted. It was nothing for which one had to be ashamed especially after it came to be known there were students who had taken five years to be accepted. Carl Fritze was one. On the surface of things, Fritze seemed an ideal candidate. He had attended Stanford University and had taken more than his share of subjects needed for a medical background. He was a middleweight boxer there, and had come from a medical family background. Candidates from Yale, Harvard, Brown and especially Stanford were often considered ahead of others because of the prestigious nature of those elite schools. It was not the case with Fritze. He was indentured to the microbiology department for a year until he was considered ready to be a first year medical student. In retrospect, the delay likely had its origins in an attitude problem of entitlement. Fritze was very competitive and had rancor for most of his younger classmates. He was disgruntled because he had been held out a year. Kaminski, with his shy asocial ways, often was the object of Fritze's antagonism, but they had something in common that had to do with being alienated from others.

Fritze and Kaminski worked hard in medical school and while Kaminski got honors in psychiatry and obstetrics, Fritze rose to the academic level that provided him with the medical honorary, Alpha Omega Alpha. He went on to become a surgeon whose practice assumed the devotion of a martyr. He became the chief of staff of his hospital, participated in professorial medical school duties which involved teaching residents. He accepted honors and was a member of many professional societies. He could be seen at all hours, on any holiday, not just attending to his patients but nursing them back to health. He lived, ate and drank his profession. When the rare occasion allowed him to socialize at a cocktail party, when asked what he did for a living, with a sneer that began and ended the conversation, a no-nonsense reply announced he was just a surgeon.

As Kaminski moved on in his life so did Fritze, until they retired about the same time. Kaminski, on the one hand, was like his polymorphous-interest addicted father. He was able to explore and enjoy multiple subjects outside of medicine for many years. He got that way for another reason; he rode no chariot, wore no laurel celebrating his triumph as a medical doctor. On the other hand, Fritze died suddenly just a year after he had retired.

Why did Fritze die shortly after retirement and Kaminski did not? Let us take stock in a different perspective than the usual explanation of death as a specific illness of the body, such as a familial susceptibility to cardiovascular disease or exposure to a specific carcinogen. Ponder instead an alternative in which their lengths of survival had something to do with different degrees of self-identity. In an antiquated way of appreciating an alternative causation of death, it can be said that Fritze died of a broken heart; he broke down and outright died when he felt he ceased to be who he thought he was. His physical death most likely followed a psychic death that was tied to his retirement. Retirement in his emotional brain eliminated an all important component of his self-identity that was defined by his most achieved status in his culture. Having nothing to live for is the sentiment of too many humans put out to pasture.

What I am saying is the reptilian emotional part of the brain to which the mind has access, has a profound effect on survival of the body. There is an ongoing day to day appreciation of the emotional status of being healthy, in good shape, happy, whatever you like. The mind as a spokesman attempts to reveal superficially that status in daily greeting with others with the simple reply: "Oh, I'm fine, thanks." to the question: "How are you, today?". In the ongoing assessment of what the mind thinks about its state of being happy, it is listening especially to the *neuroceptive* coming from the depth of its primitive emotional brain component derived from the ancient reptile. That emotional aspect of our self-identity has a simple mentality of basing its happiness, really a great deal of our homeostatis on the schemes of hierarchical dominance. Feeling good or bad has its origins in this basic, ancient, most primal emotion. So when we feel low, sad, down and out, these feelings are very often in the context of our status in the hierarchy of others, but what hierarchy, what others? Here it becomes important to see how a culture or a society plays a defining role in our self-identity because this primary emotion of feeling good (happy) or bad (depressed) is often determined by it and the groups within it.

THE CULTURAL HIERARCHY

The premise is held that the human nervous system and its derived behavior have evolved from an earlier, more primitive reptilian brain and we, therefore, retain a certain character of behaving that is typical of reptiles. We follow a genetic survival formulation of our animal ancestry. Like simple reptiles, we humans continue to exhibit a hierarchical system of dominance of our societal members. There are powerful leaders or groups and a sub-system of graduated less powerful subjects. We have a method of reproduction among the sexes that is dominated by the positions of power. Humans have a means of procuring sustenance that also follows hierarchical dominance of its members from eating in food lines to elite restaurants. Like reptiles, humans possess a given territory varying in size from country, state, county, social club, neighborhood or playground. All these territories are protected by a supreme commander of its members from intruder-predators and has been abstracted into "the laws and mores of the particular land-holding.

Now, all cultures are not the same, but each has the basic organization of its animal origins. The genetic driven undercarriage gets attached to the different values of cultures because members of each culture get a hardhat schooling of attaching the basement of the reptile's establishment to the superstructure of what the culture believes in and stands for. Each newborn babe gets its specialized cultural identification this way and those values eventually are held not as an intellectual pastime of contemplation but with the zeal of lethal defiance.

An example is the different values of pagan societies and those that acquired a Christian character after them. Native American tribal societies held it to be in their survival interests to have many gods and many wives, while just the opposite held for the Spanish settlers whose values were dominated by their Catholic teachings. Both pre-Christian and Christian societies worked from the same reptilian script of survival; both utilized the hierarchical dominance schemes of control in a given territory. Both types of societies demonstrated many of their values concerning the survival script were in great opposition which resulted in hatred and war. The Nez Pierce child of the 1870's as well as the offspring of contemporary displaced Palestinians, have had to learn the emotional value of territory and its impact on survival. Darwin's thesis was correct not just for other animal species, but for human cultures as well, because it turns out that there is an ongoing chaotic war of survival of the fittest to determine what set of values attached to the old reptilian formula will prevail.

While defining status and values of its members is inherent and obligatory in either a primitive or advanced culture, the process of acquiring a cultural status can have adverse health consequences for two fundamental reasons: 1) An individual may falter, not advance through the self-identity stages humans must pass in their maturation into cultural autonomy. This kind of impasse can even occur when an individual erringly considers his self-identity rests wholly upon the last and most noteworthy, culturally accepted status. 2) He may die from self-inflicted emotional distress along with other members when he feels his culture has come to an end due to attempts at genocide and other similar calamities.

We must not forget that self-identity is a continuum of an individual's lifelong attempt at maintaining survival, life against death. There is a cultural continuum of maintaining its survival that affects those within it. When those members of a given culture defy acculturation or it becomes apparent there is a systematic attempt to destroy their culture, there is ample evidence that a self (identity) inflicted demise can take place. This point is accurately stated as a lethal form of cultural shock by Francis Huxley in his description of the fate of Brazilian Indian tribes forced to accept the values of their Portuguese conquerors. "Nearly all Indian tribes, once pacified, succumb . . . to the two stools of their own morality (cultural value system) and the morality . . . of the Brazilians (Portuguese), they die from the despair of not being anything in particular."*

Illness and even death due to an inability to be a card carrying member in good status of a society and to move up the ladder of the accepted categories of status defined by the culture, has a patchwork history of investigation that first followed the old line of reasoning that the mind was something different than the body, but the mind had something to do with the health of the body. There were the Socratic Greeks that tied a sound mind to a sound body. There were Freudian thoughts about a "death instinct" and Hutschneckers's appreciation of the relationship between body disease and a defect in coping described in his book, *The Will to Live*. There are many other references to physical death and inexplicable mental causality; people with diseases or even healthy individuals are capable of wishing for or predicting their physical death without any logical organic explanation. In almost any family history, attention can be drawn to the peculiar closeness of time of death between long or deeply emotionally bound married couples and chronically diseased patients and their care givers. The association between mental status and illness was championed over one hundred years ago with the emergence of the field of "psychosomatic medicine", but it has been somewhat lost in the science of neurotransmission of mental disease. The relationship of illness occurring after different emotional stresses tied to disruption of various kinds of group involvement was documented by the psychiatrist, Thomas Holmes, fifty years ago. We can also see that mind-body connection in the practices of Voodoo and black magic and in Vedic Hinduism in which a wife has no cultural identity without a living husband. There are contemporary East Indian ladies that still do not shirk their duty by climbing on the funerary pyres of their departed husbands. Perhaps, the myth of Sir Galahad dying after acquiring the Holy Grail still serves as an explanation of having nothing more for which to live.

In today's medical obsession with microbiologic and genetic explanations of disease, the obvious contemporary pursuit of the mind-brain-body relationship to disease comes out of the psychiatric school of "Object Relations".** The germinal core of this discipline, while not

---

* Parentheses are this author's.

** "Object Relations: Theory and Practice" by Michael H. Horne, M.D., Grand rounds of psychiatry and behavioral sciences at the University of Washington School of Medicine, April 12, 2006.

concerned with body diseases and the mind, establishes that mental diseases are brought about because of disturbed relationships with others, (individual objects or group objects). Drawing on this psychoanalytic awareness, we can see how faulty relationships with groups proscribed to be the norm in any culture can occur and create disease.

The groups within and conforming to the overall greater ethos of a society have to do with the basic expected status a human must achieve in childhood, adolescence, and maturity. The individual must negotiate passage through these age-appropriate groups to have a group sense of self and to be a successful member of society. This format, especially for western cultures, provides a personal sense of well-being. To feel "good" an individual acquires a sense of happiness by participating as an active member of each status level. In simple terms, you feel good and secure when you are a member of those groups the culture supports. Only the rare individual, such as the outcast monk living in a cave, can sustain his survival outside of the security of his cultural domain. In this instance, the domain is not of the physical world but a spiritual one.

A culture is a large hierarchical group of individuals that interrelate with sub-hierarchies, a few members at the top and the majority providing a bottom. Once again, it must be brought to mind this arrangement has an ancient survival origin. We have established that reptiles best demonstrate the fundamental nature of this kind of animal behavior, even though more primitive animal species such as fish and some animals without backbones reveal this organizing character. Ancient cultures were defined by just a few categories of status: chief, warriors, squaws and children. In the modern western culture, there are a myriad of hierarchical groups that don't necessarily relate specifically to the overall organization of the culture. There are all the cultural identities that relate to skills, occupations and recreational interests dictated as appropriate for each level of maturation. These groups all organize in their particular territories with a distribution of membership shaped like a pyramid. Humans acquire a significant degree of self-identity by defining themselves as participating members of not only the large culture, but as members of groups within. For example, the gentleman next to you on your return flight home from Dallas gets his identity straightened out for you, a total stranger. By identifying his acceptable memberships, he reports: "I am really married even though I don't wear a wedding ring; I have five children all in private schools; I am president of the local American Legion and the California chapter of consulting flight engineers. Oh, yes, I love living in the L.A. Palisades because it has a large branch of the Church of Scientology. By the way, I am a social democrat. And who are you?"

Humans seek mental and physical security in hierarchical groups as part of their evolutionary biologic make-up to survive. One has only to envision a gaggle of snow geese rising in unison and flying away as a single entity or to watch a school of anchovies all together dart away from a predator, to understand that hierarchical groups with their distant animal origins provide a better chance of survival. Humans, it appears, cannot exist without groups either, but the survival advantage of them is not without its drawbacks when it comes to acquiring a survival-successful self-identity.

The human survival advantage of group membership is not accessed with a free pass, because the group-society itself is internally competitive with a series of proscribed steps that must be traveled to become a full member. The human flock is forever being graded, measured as to the relative position of its members. Humans also inflict their needs of measuring for the hierarchy on those domesticated animal in their keeping with blue ribbons and other signs of achievement. This endless behavior of competition, of rank, of best, the grading of performance of all variety, the very fiber of human life is hardly thought of as an emotion, yet it is the most primary feeling state of our animal natures that thrives on dominance. We suspend the failure of achievement in an abstraction called depression and other physical or mental illness not knowing of its true origins.

When an individual becomes a casualty as Fritze was, Object Relations theory explains that "it is experienced as a death of the self which if it progresses leads to a process of mourning with symptoms of sadness, meaninglessness and anxiety." And now the nexus between depression and a depressed immune system that becomes a harbinger of death and disease can be established. In the final chapter, it will come to our attention that the long-standing history of the belief of mental illness causing physical illness called psychosomatic disease is now appreciated as a new field of scientific medicine called Psycho-Neuro-Micro-immunity. For now, it is only necessary to understand that the reptilian emotional element of the central nervous system has a way of shutting down the body-brain under extreme stress. Robert Sapolsky of Stanford University School of Medicine describes how stress that is now observed to come from faulty relationships can cause or contribute to physical and mental afflictions ranging from heart disease, ulcers and memory loss to infertility and even diminished growth.

The fact that there is a link between Alzheimer's disease and depression comes as a shock to some who consider it purely a neurological disease. Because it occurs so often in older individuals, it has been tossed to the side as just a manifestation of aging, just like the disease, Senile Macular

Degeneration of the eye. However, each disease has risk factors that are not directly age related. Think about causation of Alzheimer's disease through a different port; one that would be correlated with aging, but may well have a self-identity psychic component. With this reexamination, we can use object relations theory to explain further the disease. Depression, remember, is really what the observers of object relations theory call the ultimate stress to an individual. People like Fritze become depressed when their role in society is dispatched to the bone yard. They become relics of the fireside and the wards of their mates who often are very troubled with their presence there. The depression of being an emotional nobody creates a circumstance rife with the disrespect given to a child sitting around the house. Mums and Dads once had to say to them as children, "go outside and play; get out from under my feet." The depression is heightened by more loss of self in the marital relationship as the self is given back to the mom or dad-mate. Like the Amazonian Indians Huxley observed, the brain shuts down, initiated by the deep emotional part of the human core sense of self that doesn't know who it is anymore. The problem of illness has heretofore been appreciated primarily as a manifestation of the flesh and its micro-immune system, but we can now appreciate there are these definite connections of the mind to the micro-immune system. Depression from alienation and exclusion is the emotional state that ignites this still poorly understood relationship.

Fritze provides an example of what appears to be a secure sense of self-identity from a successful object relations transit in his culture. Yet the culture may not have all the answers to self-identity. Remember the Nazis, the Romans, and the Confederates of the United States. Of even greater importance are the many individuals who fail to advance through the most significant stages of early object relations between parents and family. The illnesses that come from these primary stages of cultural involvement are, for the most part, derived from the vaults of unconscious behavior generated by the silent right hemisphere, the part of the brain attached to the emotions formed by childhood dependency relationships with others. Many mental and or physical illnesses come about because the families, the parents, and the other caregivers of the developing emotional child inculcate a faulty brand of cultural values regarding advancing through these early stages of passage. Individuals thus instructed with their off-center values of hierarchical-group survival are outcasts to the norms of status acceptance. Look at this not too obvious, but significant example. Mark, a nice young man to look at, was unfortunate enough by birth to get involved in a defective parenting strategy in which his mother was struggling with her demons to be in charge of her husband rather than accepting him as an equal partner.

(A couple is the smallest representation of the basic animal hierarchy.) Unable to dominate her husband, she focused her attention on her first son in which her object relationship with him became one of control rather than nurturing for masculine independence. Consequently, he turned out to be a "mamma's boy". He could never acquire a real male identity of independence but remained dependent upon his mother to the extent that he could not participate successfully in male organizations run by males or even in a pair-bond with a female other than his mother. He was known as the "whipping boy" to the men in his cultural groups; he acted out in passive-aggressive displays that were certain to inspire rejection. It was impossible for him to have any insight regarding his failure to fit in any group and his life-long formula resulted in his being an outcast in society. He could only persist as a ward of his mother who was forced to take him back into the defective custody of their original object relation tragedy because of his physical and mental illness. A notable exception I can recall of this faulty maturation where there was still a successful participation in the culture was the prolonged mother-son bond of Douglas MacArthur that continued even beyond his years at West Point where his mother remained in residence there to direct his behavior from a nearby hotel. Perhaps she appreciated she had a problem on her hands and it would take a lifetime of support of an unusual genius for him to make it to the top of the cultural ladder.

As we squirm with contempt at those group participants whose hair is orange and clothing black, at the political party that represents an opposing view, at the masses who provide devotion to a particular soccer team composed of foreigners, let us not forget that those attachments to groups keep humans, some of whom must do the dirty work of the culture, from going crazy. Yet, gangs are groups that alienate the culture and do not meld into it. We can see that this kind of attachment of first generation American youth to violent criminal groups is understandable because they are caught between the culture and values of their parents who do not speak English, dress and act differently in the new culture which does not easily accept them nor does it allow them to integrate into it fully. Gang membership provides these disenfranchised young people a sense of belonging to a new "family". Americans are learning that hard core gang members are not rehabilitated in our prisons which just reinforce gang life alienation. Doing "time" is a badge of distinction for advancement in the gang hierarchy.

Unfortunately, a human's concept of itself is not automatically achieved. It must successfully mature by negotiating early simple relationships to more complex ones that the culture defines in its best interests. These relationships are first very emotional with tastes and other primitive appreciations of mother, then mother and father, then siblings, then family and then other social and skill groups and eventually groups that make up adult status. As previously discussed, an individual must be well grounded through a process of interaction with others to acquire modulated emotional components to his character. Most other mammalian species acquire self-identity quickly within a simplistic group arrangement, the pride or the troupe. The human, on the other hand, must mature by passing through a number of groups that are critical to becoming relatively independent. Human self-identity is not established at birth or easily acquired, but is determined by successful negotiation of many human relationships. Failures can be single events or multiple ones as a human gains mental maturity. These failures are not always obvious to behold or evident in the transfer from one earlier group to a more advanced one. The fallout may occur when a secure adult cultural status seems achieved. (Post partum psychosis falls into this concept when the realization of being a mother creates the loss of a former self-identity. By the same token, some women become distraught when becoming a mother can not be achieved.) However, the lack of evidence of failure is often provided by the dualistic nature of the human brain in which the dark side is kept hidden for as long as possible. The judge who made unwanted sexual advances to his clerks in chambers is an example. The high school football hero who is unable to define himself outside of the bars of habitues that remember him is another. The twenty-seven year old stepson living with his parents and getting engaged to be married establishes the current problems of smoothly going from one cultural group to another without the proper credentials.

A moment of digression is appropriate here because it has been bantered about for these many hundreds of years that the mind has something to do with the health of the body which now includes the brain. Consequently we need to return to the second section of this book and review what happened to Freud. In that chapter, it was pointed out that he was under the gun of his contemporary scientists to establish a physical foundation of his analytical (talking cure) theory of treating mind disorders, most significantly, the hysterias. He was in a far graver situation than Pasteur who was able to debunk scientifically his antagonists who felt his theory of fermentation was a throwback to vitalist interpretations of disease. Both men were challenged because Helmholtz and others previously mentioned, appreciated the time had come where it was necessary to explain and cure disease by the new scientific methods of physical observation. Seeing the effect of bacteria on an infected organ under a microscope is a no nonsense example of their demands. "Show me the money" was the rigid requirement to remove the metaphysical gobbledygook of the past. As noted before, Freud was not able to do this even though he turned away from hypnotic treatment in an attempt to make his theory more scientific. Yet no one could find anatomically the Ego and the Id and the Super Ego or, for that matter, the subconscious that he described. Scientists today have disenfranchised Freudian and analytic treatment for this very reason. As we look back, however, it is possible now to underscore anatomically his theory with physical evidence. Freud and the past champions of the scientific method were not in a position to understand Mesmer's and Charcot's hypnotism techniques as actually having a physical neurological explanation.

Taking note of previously mentioned observations of the evolution of the left symbolic neocortex, it can be remembered that children, as well as primitive humans, learning auditory language first learn by association word symbols with objects appreciated primarily by vision but all the other senses as well, and then learn whole body movements associated with word symbols. Johnny run, sit, eat, stay; just like Bowser is able to associate certain word symbols with whole body acts. Therefore, there are neurological connections between words and complex body movements that we identified as part of the mechanism of Penfield's hippocampal—automatic motor system. In hypnotic techniques, the fundamental process is called extra-personal suggestion, a contemporary remnant of our auditory symbolic development. When we identify the mind as being the primary auditory symbolic left neo-cortex, it can be appreciated that part of the central nervous system can activate or inhibit by neuron synaptic processing, body acts. It also can be understood that through autosuggestion, such as "glove anesthesia" there can be a neuron derived synaptic inhibition of certain body processes so typical of hysteria otherwise known as a conversion reaction. If the two sciences of mind and brain can come together and stop thinking they are separate entities, we can accept the profound influence the mind part of the brain can have on other parts of the brain and the body. It is now accepted fact that a depressed mind can depress the immune system to the extent that physical illness can occur, yet this old primary emotion of withdrawal-defense derived from reptiles can have an acute beneficial effect when survival is out of the question.

The understanding of this acute regulation of the immune system came from the early observations of a condition that was identified by Charles R. Richet and Paul J. Portier in the early nineteenth century when they studied unexplained sensitization and deaths of laboratory animals following a second injection of antigen. The process of hypersensitivity, (over reaction) of the immune system was drastic enough to cause death of the test animals from their own defensive immune reaction. The process was called, *anaphylaxis*, a word they derived from the Greek "the lack of immunity protection". The process was initially considered one of hypersensitivity (over-reaction) of the immune system that was drastic enough to cause death of the test animals from their own defensive immune reactions. The suddenness of anaphylaxis in the human experience, often with lethal consequences, can occur from bee venom. Yet, here again, the old investigators were looking at the immune system as an isolated micro-cellular-antigen-antibody event. They did not understand that this thing they named anaphylaxis involved the nervous system as well. Over time it has come to be identified as "anaphylactic shock". This terminology more accurately acknowledges that something else happens besides excessive amounts of antigen not being blocked or being excessively blocked by an appropriate amount of antibody.

Shock is a neurological process of the central nervous system that can occur without any sign of micro-immune action or mental depression. Brain derived shock occurs profoundly when there is excessive trauma, blood loss or oxygen starvation. Another type of shock, known as a vaso-vagal reflex is not lethal and does not involve the micro-immune system but does cause an unusually frightened individual to faint at the sight of a mouse or blood, for example. This reflex involves the autonomic nervous system of fight or flight especially dealing with the vascular regulatory system of the heart. Matzinger postulates that the link between the brain and the micro-immune system occurs with the meeting of a globular T cell with a long armed danger-sensing dendritic cell. There is the current knowledge of the cellular process of *apoptosis* in which cells regulate their longevity and die so that new cells can emerge and replicate their original functions all over the body. It does not take too much of a stretch to grasp that the cells of the central nervous system especially those that include the most primitive survival emotions can also participate in this normal biologic process.

The best understanding of a mind-brain derived form of near lethal shock from fright comes from an early observation of Dr. David Livingstone written in 1850 of a lion attack.

"I heard a shout. Starting and looking half-around, I saw a lion just in the act of springing on me. I was upon a little height; he caught my shoulder as he sprang, and we both came to the ground below together. Growling horribly close to my ear, he shook me as a terrier does a rat. The shock produced a stupor similar to that which seems to be felt by a mouse after the first shake of the cat. It caused a sort of dreaminess in which there was no sense of pain nor feeling of terror, though quite conscious of all that was happening. It was like what patients partially

under the influence of chloroform describe, who see all the operation but feel not the knife. This singular condition was not the result of any mental process. The shake annihilated fear, and allowed no sense of horror in looking around at the beast. This peculiar state is probably produced in all animals killed by the carnivore; and if so, it is a merciful provision by our benevolent creator for lessening the pain of death."

Modern biologic science must come to grips with the complex effects of the emotional components of the brain on health and survival.

Chapter 9

THE SENSE OF SELF AND
MIND-BODY DISEASES

HOW MULTIPLE SCLEROSIS BECOMES A CENTRAL NERVOUS
SYSTEM DISEASE OF MIND AND BRAIN.

One fall day when the school board piped the young to return to school, David Kaminski stepped outside his parent's home to restart the drudgery. Glumly rounding the corner of his block, his attention was drawn to an unfamiliar vocal duet between a mother clad in her nightgown and a son on his way to school. With one hand she had pushed the screen door aside not to inhibit the quality of her part of the performance. Softly and sweetly with mellifluous intent she called out to her seven year old son. Hesitantly he moved away intermittently standing in stanzas of physical and emotional departure. Going in the opposite direction of Kaminski's path, the child was on the way to his first year of grade school. Each morning thereafter, the students' paths crossed; in fact, Kaminski looked forward to the strange uttering of the songbirds. He was drawn to its memory for most of his adult life for reasons he could not explain.

The duet went this way: "Love, love" said the mother; "Kiss, kiss" said the young child. On and on it went for a distance that finally took the child out of sight. The troubadourian laments diminished now, brought on a harsh critique. "The little sissy," Kaminski thought. "The little jerk, why did that mother molly-coddle him so much? What an idiot that mother was." In future recollections during nights of traveling on undivided highways or trying to sleep upright on long jet flights, the memory of that mother and child popped up in his consciousness. In time, it was always accompanied by a memory of his own childhood.

On Kaminski's way to grade school as a nine year old, his journey took him by a gas station whose attendant when not pumping gas, was inside the garage greasing cars and changing oil. A more direct route home took Kaminski not past the station, but through it, across a rubber covered wire that rang a bell for the mechanic to hear and come outside to service his gas customers' needs. What fun it was to stomp on the rubber wire and hear the same sound the bell produced when his school day came to its end! After not too many repetitions of this play, out popped the mechanic with a large wrench in his hand. "Listen, sonny boy, I am going to hit you right on your pretty little head if you step on that line one more time." The declaration was finished with a devil's grin. Tears and the rush home quivering with fright gave substance to the tale of the big, bad wolf. "Your father will be here soon, you tell him what happened." Not at all isolated from its emotional candor, the same story told again to the household authoritarian, failed to get the hoped for solution from Calvin Kaminski just home from work.

The father placed his hand on David's shoulder and said: "Next time, don't step on that rubber wire; go around it, Son." Forever remembering the account, David vowed that he would always come to his own sons' rescue. He would never be as cruel as his own father had been.

So it came to pass, David, the father of two sons, on many occasions arose to defend them with that indelible proclamation of assistance. On one occasion, he stomped into the local police station and reported a worker setting up concrete forms for new sidewalks. "That worker abused my little boy by telling him he would beat his ass if he wrote his initials in any more wet concrete. You must arrest that man." On another occasion, David Kaminski bounded from the stands onto a basketball court and bumped his chest on a dumbfounded referee for not making the right call.

One night, after his sons had grown but continued to plague him with the need to bail them out of adult responsibilities, David Kaminski awoke to an inspirational insight that his own father had done him a favor and he had done his own sons a disfavor. He clearly realized now that his sons were burdened as adults with an inability to stand up for themselves because their father was always saving them from having to do so on their own.

Modern scientific investigation appreciates human immunity is a composition of multiple disciplines. Survival against any particular disease is now understood as having psychological, neurological and micro-cellular humeral elements. The mind can influence the nervous system which, in turn, can influence the micro-immune system. In this regard, investigators consider immunity to include: 1) protection against diseases caused by microorganisms and 2) protection against large predators and competitors. The new theory of immunity known as psycho-neuro-immunity readily interfaces with the concept of human self-identity as both provide an understanding of how humans survive. While immunity once referred solely to our defenses against microscopic predators, the new concept of immunity concerns our survival and defenses against both microscopic and large predators which may include other humans. With respect to large predators, immunity is a developmental system of increasingly more complex brain components that include the mind, the auditory symbolic communication part of the brain. The development in each human is a reflection of evolution and is fraught with opportunities for defects to occur.

In the process of evolution, organisms gain more complexity as survival becomes more complex. There is an ongoing need to adapt to changes in order to survive. The need is not automatically granted to every human, every society and every culture. Certain cultures and certain individuals within those cultures have developed more successful complex strategies than others. All citizens of the United States have those constitutionally granted rights but not necessarily the survival capabilities to utilize them.

Survival against large predators includes competing successfully with humans of one's own society as well as defending against societies trying to enslave or destroy. Lawfully competing members of our society and individuals who seek to destroy us physically in criminal acts or economically in civil acts can pose a threat to our survival. Human immunity also includes defenses against all animal predators that include bears, tigers and rattlesnakes. Not so obvious immunity includes defenses that establish independence from others in socio-economic situations and even involve independence from one's own family members.

When fully developed all these immunity functions including the micro-immune element are regulated in an orderly fashion by the central nervous system. Our large predator protection is most elementary in the form of the spinal reflex against the pain of excess energy or the bite of a predator. This reflex insures a withdrawal of a given part of the body under attack. Just above the spinal reflex, in the midbrain, large predator protection becomes more complex in a specific area called the "alarm center", also known as the locus ceruleus. This component is located just under the reptilian analog of the human brain. When this alarm center goes off, it alerts the rest of the brain for survival action, especially against large predators. The process results in multiple hormonal, vascular and micro-immune responses of fight or flight. The reptile's ancient responsiveness is the pivotal point between large and microscopic immunity. Higher still are the brain centers that provide more complex responses for survival that include temporary hierarchical pacifism among rivals and mates. These are functions of the limbic part of the brain. Then, at the summit of the brain within neo-cortical levels of intelligence, there are the thinking and symbolic elements of the brain, the use of which allows humans to survive by adaptation even when one society is pitted against another with more effective weapons or methods of trade or instruments of competition for goods and services. There have also occurred in the higher complexity of the cerebral cortices of the human brain, survival functions of enhanced competition among rivals within a given society. These survival functions are primarily thinking strategies that result in nonviolent negotiation and reason with associates and with family members. Hence in our society, an individual who is able to out-think, out-wit, out-guess or out-talk another is considered to have admirable qualities.

Until now, the concepts of survival and immunity have been confined to the body; the mind has not been involved. However, the precise junction of immunity of the mind and the nervous system is in an old brain structure called the hypothalamus. This structure is within the lower level of brain development called the diencephalon, the reptilian component of the human brain. Here, humeral and cellular micro-immune functions of the body are connected to the reptilian station by the autonomic nervous system. The autonomic nervous system not only regulates and protects our body and its organs but also interacts with the cells and fluids of micro-cellular immunity. The reptilian part of the brain is the pivotal point of the central nervous system immunity against large predators of other species as well as against competitors and enemies of our own kind. The reptilian nervous system element of immunity is a twofold interaction of the mind and the micro-cellular system for both large predators and microscopic invaders. Neuro-immunologists refer to this junction as the HYPAC AXIS. It is now appreciated that micro-immune functions are primarily regulated by this part of the brain. What comes as a surprise to researchers is the knowledge of the mind's effect on this system.

Single celled animals can be stimulated by a painful or stressful stimulus and can then respond to that stimulus by withdrawal. More complex multi-cellular organisms can be similarly stimulated and they can respond to the stimulus with both withdrawal and other simple survival activities. As stimuli become mixed and less painful more complex multi-cellular organisms with brains have evolved with increasingly sophisticated means of responding to stressful stimuli. The human has the greatest degree of complexity of the large animals to sense complex stimuli and react to them. This ability is derived from the human's use of auditory and visual symbolic communication in his mind.

When the complexity of a survival stimulus excites but does not cause an appropriate complex response to discharge the buildup of the excitation, the brain utilizes the next most complex response it can muster. This has been previously referred to as a *regressive immune response*. A regression occurs when a simpler, less complex response discharges the excitation of a more complex stimulus. It is as if a student were asked to play a complicated piece of music on his trumpet. Not knowing the piece, he responds by playing a much more simplistic one. Another example would be the student trying to survive an examination, who regresses to crib notes or his neighbor's paper for the answers.

An excessive build-up of excitation within a neuron or a system of neurons occurs when the most appropriate response does not occur; an electrochemical disequilibrium results. Unanswered, extended stimulation of neurons results in fatigue and eventual damage. Examples of damage are plentiful in every component of total immunity when the stress is not relieved. There is combat fatigue in the mind, nerve paresis in the brain, agranulocytosis in the micro-immune system. A regressive immune response is an important means by which the brain abrogates the stress by whatever means it has in its vertically aligned defenses. Regressive immune brain behavior provides a new way of looking at illness. Illness becomes the ultimate down-regulated response of a difficult stress. It provides for equilibrium within the nervous system through its most primitive micro-cellular element of defense. Humans get sick because there is often no other way to relieve stress. One doesn't need to look far to find multiple examples of human stresses that build up until an illness occurs. The illness provides an equilibrating reduction of the stress by a response not entirely appropriate. It is a down-regulation, a regression going back to more primitive means of releasing stress. Illness can be a good thing, but not on an ongoing, recurring basis. Then it can become lethal in the form of a chronic unchecked disease.

The human ego defense mechanisms which may employ illness (withdrawal) as a relief from stress are survival behaviors carried over from the reptilian mandate. Ego defense mechanisms are aptly named but misunderstood as being associated solely with a type of reasoning present only in neurotic-psychotic minds. Actually, ego defenses represent an ancient form of thinking that humans are trying to put behind them in the complex process of evolution. Contemporary humans who continue to utilize only thinking processes we call ego defense mechanisms (making excuses, blaming, attacking others verbally, projecting, sulking, withdrawing) against more sagacious individuals, can be considered to possess an older, once appropriate, way of thinking that now is a defective form of immunity. Individuals who have less adequate survival strategies against human rivals and competitors can bring about serious social-psychological consequences. The consequences are also serious with respect to germs, the small predators. It is not greatly appreciated that defective mind and other less developed brain components of immunity against large predators can result in activation of the micro-immune system. Depression can actually adversely affect our lymph cells that fight germs. There is also evidence that unresolved stress in dealing with others can cause defects in the regulation of the micro-immune system which result in autoimmune diseases. The defective ways of managing stress also cause the difficult to explain variations in human susceptibility to microbiological insults. For instance, an individual having sex with another who is diseased with syphilis has a 50% chance of acquiring the disease, not a 100% chance. The odds making the possibility more likely are related to personality types and their specific kinds of mind-directed behavior. Certain psychological types of gay men have been shown to respond to HIV treatment better than other types. Additionally, a study from Boston University found decreased micro-immunity in children that were poorly nurtured in foster homes. Our inattention to the mind and central nervous system actions in immunity comes from a long history of study by scientists just trying to understand immunity's microscopic character. Scientific thinking began as a study of blood-borne cellular and humeral defenses against germs. However, the studies cited above, along with an increasing number of others point to the mind as being instrumental in immunity or a lack thereof.

THE TRIPARTITE IMMUNE REGRESSION MODEL: MULTIPLE SCLEROSIS

This enigmatic disease has only been appreciated by medical science as a disease of the micro-immune component of immunity. Attention has been entirely focused on what goes on at the humeral-cellular level; the mechanism of T cells of the immune system attacking myelin. In the self-identity (psycho-neuro-immunity) concept, multiple sclerosis can be understood as a disease also of mind and brain immunity against large predators. The disease involves all three components: mind, brain and micro-cellular immune system. In multiple sclerosis, like so many other diseases, a marginally developed mind that defectively competes or that meets a life situation in which it cannot compete, causes stress with unrelenting stimulation of the HYPAC AXIS of the nervous system which, in turn, continues to stimulate the micro-immune system in an abnormal manner.

Mind stress regardless of its content activates the old reptilian neuro-system of survival, fight or flight until the stress is eliminated. In humans, the fight-flight system is connected to the micro-immune system that takes part in the survival mechanism. (When reptiles fought or ran away, it was almost always associated with a body injury. The cellular and humeral mechanisms of survival were always called upon to take care of body injuries.) Social stresses don't cause body injury from combat, but they still activate on a lesser scale all the mechanisms that were once needed to stop infections and heal wounds. MS patients do not solve social-competitive stress with just a regressive mind response, the neuro-mechanism of fight or flight or just a body-illness response, but a combination of all three. The MS patient is a prototype of what happens in chronic disease, especially cancer and lethal forms of collagen diseases we consider autoimmune. In multiple sclerosis, unabated mind stress often associated with neurotic dependency hammers the HYPAC AXIS that inherently involves the micro-immune system.

The MS genetically respondent or predisposed person has an inability to solve ordinary stresses with appropriate responses most of us enjoy. As stresses accumulate, they are not solved with reason and negotiation, nor with neurotic or addictive behavior. The patient feels trapped and down-regulation or regression of his survival mechanisms occurs even further. The MS patient often down-regulates his solutions by default with respect to mind solutions, because he was never given the chance to develop them fully. He, like other unsuccessful individuals, essentially tries to compete in adulthood with childhood dependency strategies that lack independence of action and decisiveness. In many cases, the MS patient may appear to be a dominant authority figure in charge of others in corporations, in friendships and in the family, but he is not truly an independent thinker. He controls much as a child tries to control his parents by mimicking early parental directives, or with other learned behaviors such as, temper tantrums, sulkiness, moodiness, argumentative behavior or despondent helplessness. Minds with regressive or undeveloped states of dependency do not relieve stress in the adult world, but continue to create it. Unrelieved stresses caused by dependent behavior continue to down regulate the survival system by activating the neurological (reptilian brain) of fight or flight. The excessive unrelenting stimulation of the neurological mechanism, the HYPAC AXIS in the hypothalamus, does not result in a cold or the flu, but in a chronic autoimmune disease like systemic lupus erythematosus. Like many autoimmune diseases that involve blood vessels, MS specifically is to be considered an end-arterial vascular illness of cerebral blood vessels. The vasculopathy does not occur in the vessels of the heart to cause heart attacks or in the peripheral vascular bed to cause hypertension, but like a stroke, it occurs in a finite genetically susceptible segment of brain circulation known as a pre-capillary arteriole. The sustained insult eventually results in focal brain infarction and plaque formation. The micro-elements of immunity are activated in the form of specialized white corpuscles drawn to the injury site. In curious, unremitting cases, they are unable to clear the damage to the brain or to the mind of the MS patient. Consequently, there is plaque formation.

The characteristic term to describe the mind state of the MS patient is *belle indifference*. This refers to observations in which patients are considered "unusually euphoric", "absurdly cheerful" and toward the end, as Charcot penned, "to possess stupid indifference to all things". Rather than be considered cognitive dysfunctions secondary to the disease, these mind characteristics are to be considered part of a defective self-identity mind disorder that *predates* the onset of the neurological damage and continues afterwards. The defective mind disorder falls into the category of neurotic behavior of excessive dependency associated with an illness. The *belle indifference* characteristic of MS and other chronic diseases, for the most part, involves a real illness. Individuals with *belle indifference* often have an ongoing disease about which they are not really depressed or appropriately concerned.

In 1940, Sir Russel Brain described the *belle indifference of MS* as a mental disorder of dissociation known as a *conversion reaction* or *hysteria*. (In this mind condition, there is a separation of certain thoughts or body processes from an individual's conscious awareness. A patient will be separated in his thinking from memories, emotional states or parts of his body and, most importantly, from diseases of his body.) Sir Russel Brain recognized that this mind disease was a fundamental companion of the neurological disease of MS.

When a serious regressive immune response in a chronic disease occurs, the poorly adapted dependent mind unconsciously sees the illness as a solution to stress. These dissociation reactions are florid in individuals who have not developed an independent thinking mind or who feel that their given situation in life prevents independent action. The mental process of being unable to recognize a disease in the body or remember a traumatic event starts out in more adequate people as a mental process of voluntary denial. Psycho-neurological dissociation is a more profound state of unconscious involuntary separation characteristic of less evolved humans from the past. The MS patient unconsciously relieves stress through the regressive neurological process of becoming physically ill. His mind eliminates *external* stresses with the excuse of illness, but the stresses of life continue as *internal* stresses of the maladaptation of dependency. The mind of a dependent person, childlike, can't find solutions with independent action even as rudimentary as flight or fight. His mind ruminates, worries about others upon whom he is dependent. He is in a childlike pattern of trying to control those upon whom he is dependent. The process only causes more stress; ask any caregiver involved in control conflicts with his patient. The internal stresses continue to drive the HYPAC AXIS with damaging spastic fight or flight constriction of precapillary brain arterioles. Once hypoxia to the neurons due to circulatory injury occurs, the T cells of the micro-immune system respond to the damaged brain cells. The long-term cure of this debilitating disease rests on its prevention through recognition of its entire scope of causality from environmental, genetic, developmental, physiological, and psychological factors. The immediate direction neurobiologists must take to help those afflicted is to identify specific organic chemical substances to block the hypoxic effects of spastically attenuated precapillary arterioles in the brain. In the meantime, the inuring of an integrated sense of self by everyone responsible for the care and raising of our young is paramount to the future of man lest he succumb to disease and extinction in this increasingly stressful world.

Epilog

Through the discourse of this book, it is evident that the human brain in its evolution lost the absolute bilateral symmetry characteristic of earlier vertebrates and invertebrates. That brain evolution is ongoing and human behavior driven by it, leaves in its wake not an obvious step by step uniformity, but behaviors characteristic of lesser brain forms of other animal species. Modern colloquialisms describe behavior outside of the society's standards as asocial, defective, bi-polar, schizophrenic or criminal. The defective behaviors can be identified in this evolutionary perspective as throwbacks to earlier forms of man and his forbears. This orientation requires a renewed look at Lamarck's awareness that newborn brains, indeed all of their physical maturation, must perilously recapitulate the progressive stages of the evolution of life itself to become fully human. Kaminski and his family members and many of the anecdotes regarding his medical associates and friends point to the subtle variations of so called "normal" behaviors that are actual evidence of defective and incomplete maturation. A "normal" human is easy to recognize by physical morphology and by rudimentary language usage, but subtle developmental abnormalities are obscured by that language. It is paramount to recall the asymmetry of the human brain resulted in a dualistic world of sensory perception first associated with visual symbols and then auditory ones in which the human could experience a virtual reality without actually being there first hand. Conversely, it provided defective social humans the capability to deceive, not to be held accountable for their actions, and to operate with a morbid schizoid self-identity.

The evolution of an asymmetrical brain with one half of the cerebral cortex capable of creating language symbols marked the "end of Eden" and begot a human consciousness that could inhibit animal-emotional behavior expressed by the other half of the cerebral cortex. The asymmetry of the brain's cerebral cortex resulted in one part that produced symbolic verbal and visual control which many still refer to as the "word of God" or a "sign from God". This civilizing process had its historical roots in the mandates of monotheism. Religious leaders seized upon the teachings of their prophets and preached that God's will was to curb mankind's animal behavior and base emotions as a necessity for large numbers of humans living together. However, it came to the attention of many great thinkers who came later that the humanizing process in which control by the auditory-visual symbolic half of the brain over the other emotional-animal behavior side of the brain was excessive, even dehumanizing. Some have called it a psychosis of culture (Gooch), doomed to failure (Spengler), and a discontent of culture (Freud). These men believed that the inhibition of emotions had not taken the desired course and mankind was psychotic, discontented or doomed because of the repression of his emotions. Nevertheless, all the detractors of the effects of excessive emotional suppression would be surprised to note that current modern societies are not going crazy from too much suppression of our animal natures but too little inhibition of them.

The adverse effects of cultural evolution are to be appreciated in this book from a neurobiologic perspective. Here it has been posited that the left language brain hemisphere's inhibition of the right hemisphere dominated by the emotions is being short-circuited in modern society. While once inhibiting animal behavior by means of symbolic language, the same symbols, through visual and auditory technology, are creating an alienation of one half of the brain from the other by just the opposite effect, little suppression and a reversion to earlier animal behavior. The transposition results in poor maturation of the brain on a grand scale. As Stanley Greenspan defines, "cultural failure comes from the impoverished human awareness that human brains must mature in a process that stimulates and regulates the emotions of love and hate." As in the cited case of autism in Kaminski's family or any family with autistic children, Greenspan particularly notes the lack of this kind of emotional regulation.

In addition, no one in this day and age of microbiologic understanding of disease has thought of MS as a developmental disease. Newborn human brains must obligatorily recapitulate the evolution of mankind to remain on track for survival. If not so accomplished, the symbolic appreciating half of the central nervous system is in a state of schizophrenic dissociation from its body-needs appreciating half.

As cultures grow in their technological accomplishments, which are considered a measure of their seemingly successful survival, many leaders of these cultures fail to appreciate that the technological success may be shortsighted in the long run, if the symbolic content does not provide the need to control animal-emotional behavior in a healthy manner. I have attempted to define what is happening neurologically in the poorly matured brain-mind that is causing increasingly stressful dissociation that results in physical disease and social incompatibility. Without a complete maturation, especially with regard to the regulation of the basic emotions of love and hate as well as the development of competitive skills, cultures and individuals within them fail to survive. The flight to the virtual world of scientific symbolic invention that deals with violence and unregulated love and disregard for human relations is coming to be the norm. What could possibly be wrong with the sight of two young mothers walking side by side down a busy San Francisco avenue, not talking to each other but to far distant individuals on their cell phones, while their children are reared in affective deprived day care centers by video games and other entertainment that provide no emotional grounding? The answer has profound survival consequences.

M. K. J.

Notes

PART I: A BRIEF DESCRIPTION OF THE EVOLUTIONARY EVENTS THAT LED TO HUMAN SELF-IDENTITY.

INTRODUCTION

xi   Frishberg, Manny. "A Seattle Institute Picks Up Where the Genome Project Left Off." *Seattle Metropolitan* July 2006: 52

xi   Senet, Andre. *Man In Search of His Ancestors*. New York: McGraw Hill, 1955.

xi   Teilhard de Chardin, Pierre. *The Phenomenon of Man*. New York: Harper Row, 1959.

xii   Delacato, Carl H. *The Diagnosis and Treatment of Speech and Reading Problems*. Springfield, Illinois: Chase Thomas Company, 1964.

xii-xiii   Hayman, Ronald. *A Life of Jung*. New York, London: W. W. Norton and Company, 1999. 30-31.

xiii   Hofstadter, Douglas R. and Dennett, Daniel C., editors. *The Mind's "I"*. (Regarding Morowitz and Slobodkin) New York, Toronto: Bantam Books, 1982.

xiii   Gooch, Stan. *Total Man*. New York: Ballantine Books, 1974.

xiii   Laing, R. D. *The Divided Self*. New York: Pantheon Books, 1960.

CHAPTER 1: THE LAND OF OZ

2   Foch, Ferdinand. *The Principles of War*. London: Chapman and Hall, 1921.

3-4   Sigal, Leonard H. and Ron, Yacov. *Immunology and Inflammation*. New York: McGraw Hill, Inc., 1994

4   Buchsbaum, Ralph. *Animals Without Backbones*. Chicago: Chicago Press, 1948.

CHAPTER 2: THE REPTILE EXPANDS ITS SENSE OF SELF

8-9   Tinbergen, M. *The Study of Instinct*. Oxford: The Clarendon Press, 1951.

9   Lorenz, Konrad. *On Aggression*. New York: Harcourt, Brace and World, Inc., 1966.

9   MacLean, Paul D. "Brain Function and Socio-Sexual Behavior" from *Contemporary Sexual Behavior Critical Issues in the 1970's*. Zubin, Joseph and Money, John, editors. Baltimore: Johns Hopkins University Press, 1973.

CHAPTER 3: OLD MAMMAL CHANGES IN THE REPTILIAN SENSE OF SELF

13   Romer, Alfred Sherwood. *Man and the Vertebrates*. Chicago: University of Chicago Press, 1948.

CHAPTER 4: PRIMATE MANAGEMENT OF OLD MAMMALIAN MECHANISMS OF SELF

18-19   Collins, Treacher F. *Arboreal Life and the Evolution of the Human Eye*. Philadelphia: Lea and Febiger, 1922.

18-19   Shastid, Thomas. *Our Own and Our Cousins' Eyes*. Southbridge, Mass: American Optical Company Publication, 1926.

CHAPTER 5: THE MODEL H

23   Wilbur, Ken. *Up From Eden*. Boulder, Colorado: Shambhala Press, 1983.

25   White, Ann Terry. *Men Before Adam*. New York: Random House, 1942.

25   Wilbur, Ken. re: Levy-Bruhl and Taylor in *Up From Eden*. Boulder, Colorado: Shambhala Press, 1983.

26   Sorenson, Roger, M.D. "Dissertation on Clan Ego".

25-26   West, Willis. *The Ancient World*. Boston: Allyn and Bacon, 1913.

CHAPTER 6: A FEMALE VOICE IN THE ANCIENT WILDERNESS

28   West, Willis. *The Ancient World*. Boston: Allyn and Bacon, 1913.

28   Hinde, R. A, *Non-Verbal Communication*. Cambridge, Mass: The University Press, 1972.

29-31   Fisher, Helen. "Science of the Sexes" Discovery Channel Documentary. Discovery.com Jan. 16, 2003.

29   Jaynes, Julian. *The Origin of Consciousness in the Break-Down of the Bicameral Mind*. Boston, Mass.: Houghton Mifflin Company, 1976.

29   Wilbur, Ken. re: Arieti and Sullivan in *Up From Eden*. Boulder, Colorado: Shambhala Press, 1983.

30   Sorenson, Roger, M.D. "Dissertation on Clan Ego".

CHAPTER 7: TO BE OR NOT TO BE

36   Jaynes, Julian. *The Origin of Consciousness in the Break-Down of the Bicameral Mind*. Boston, Mass: Houghton Mifflin Company, 1976.

36   Aries, Philippe and Duby, Georges, general editors. *A History of Private Life*. "The Practical Impact of Writing" pages 111-159 by Roger Chartier. Cambridge Mass: Belknap Press, 1989.

37   Wibur, Ken. re: Piaget and Hall in *Up From Eden*. Boulder, Colorado: Shambhala Press, 1983.

37   Pavlov, Ivan. *Conditioned Reflexes: An Investigation of the Physiological Activity of the Cerebral Cortex*. London: Oxford University Press, 1927.

37-38 Aries, Phillipe and Duby, Georges, general editors. *A History of Private Life*. Cambridge, Mass: Belknap Press, 1989.

38   Roberts, J. M. *The New History of the World*. re: German culture New York: Oxford University Press, 2003.

CHAPTER 8: THE EVOLUTION OF THINKING

40-41 Ranson, Stephen and Clark, Sam. *Anatomy of the Nervous System*. Philadelphia: B. W. Saunders Co., 1953.

41-42 Aries, Philippe and Duby, Georges, general editors. *A History of Private Life*. Cambridge, Mass: Belknap Press, 1989.

42-43 Wells, H. G. *The Outline of History*. Chapter XVI "Writing" New York: MacMillan Company, 1921.

44   Bloom, Benjamin S. *All Our Children Learning*. New York: McGraw-Hill, 1980.

45   Damasio, Antonio R. *Descartes' Error*. New York: Avon Books, 1994.

45   Dubos, Rene. *Pasteur and Modern Science*. New York: Anchor Books, 1960.

45   Alexander, F. M.D. and Selesnick, S. M.D. re: Jung. in *The History of Psychiatry*. New York: Harper and Row, 1966.

PART II: A BRIEF HISTORY OF HUMAN THOUGHTS ABOUT HUMAN NATURE

INTRODUCTION

50   Henig, Robin Marantz. *Monk in the Garden: The Lost and Found Genius of Gregor Mendel, the Father of Genetics*. Boston: Houghton Mifflin, 2000.

51   Klinger, Eric. *The Structure and Function of Fantasy*. New York: Wiley Interscience, 1971.

51   Ingles, Brian. *A History of Medicine*. Cleveland, Ohio: The World Publishing Company, 1965.

51   Brentano, Franz. *Descriptive Psychology*. transl. by Benito Muller. London: Routledge, 1995.

CHAPTER 1: THE SPIRIT IS BORN

54   Romer, Alfred Sherwood. *Man and the Vertebrates*. Chicago: University of Chicago Press, 1948.

54   White, Ann Terry. *Men Before Adam.* New York: Random House, 1942.

55   West, Willis M. *The Ancient World.* Boston: Allyn and Bacon, 1913.

56   Stenhouse, T.B.H. *The Rocky Mountain Saints.* New York: Appleton and Company, 1873.

CHAPTER 2: THE HOUSES OF GODS

59   Stenhouse, T.B.H. *The Rocky Mountain Saints.* New York: Appleton and Company, 1873.

60   Toynbee, Arnold (Joseph). *A Study of History Volume I: Introduction; The Geneses of Civilization.* Oxford: Oxford University Press, 1934.

60   Mitchener, James. *Hawaii.* New York: Random House, 1959

62   Campbell, Joseph. "Myths To Live By" *Bill Moyers Journal.* 1981.

62   West, Willis. *The Ancient World.* Boston: Allyn and Bacon, 1913.

63   Coleman, James C. *Abnormal Psychology and Modern Life.* Chicago: Scott Foresman and Company, 1984.

CHAPTER 3: BODY OVER MIND

66   Netter, Frank H., M.D. "The Nervous System" *The Ciba Collection of Medical Illustration. Vol. 1.* New York: Ciba Pharmaceutical Company, 1979.

66   Sorenson, Roger M.D. Personal communication.

66-67 Ingles, Brian. *A History of Medicine.* Cleveland, Ohio: The World Publishing Company, 1965.

67   Coleman, James C. *Abnormal Psychology and Modern Life.* Chicago: Scott Foresman and Company, 1984.

68   Haldane, E. S. and Ross, G. R. T. *The Philosophical Works of Descartes.* Cambridge Mass: The Cambridge University Press, 1967.

69-70 Porter, R. *The Greatest Benefit to Mankind: A Medical History of Humanity from Antiquity to the Present.* Yew York: Harper Collins, 1997.

70   Dubos, Rene Jules. *Pasteur and Modern Science.* New York: Anchor Books, 1960.

CHAPTER 4: TERRITORIAL IMPERATIVE

74   Durrell, Lawrence. *Caesar's Vast Ghost.* New York: Arcade Publishing, 1990.

74   Gooch, Stan. *Total Man.* New York: Ballantine Books, 1974.

75   de Camp, L. Sprague. *The Great Monkey Trial.* New York: Doubleday, 1968.

75   Darwin, Charles. *The Origin of the Species.* New York: Random House, 1979.

75-76 Altholz, Josef L. "The Huxley-Wilberforce Debate Revisited." *Journal of the History of Medicine and Allied Sciences.* 35 (1980) 313-316.

77   Freud, Sigmund. *A General Introduction to Psychoanalysis.* London: Liveright Publishing Corporation, 1924.

CHAPTER 5: THE BODY OF EVIDENCE

80   Kraepelin, Emil. *Psychiatry: A Textbook for Students and Physicians.* U.S.A.: Science History Publications, 1990.

80   Goetz, C.G., Bonduelle, M., and Gelfand, T. *Charcot: Constructing Neurology.* New York: Oxford University Press, 1995.

80   Freud, Sigmund. *Dictionary of Psychoanalysis.* Geenwich, Connecticutt: Fawcett Publications, 1958.

81   O'Donnell, J. *The Origins of Behaviorism: American Psychology, 1870-1920.* New York: NYU Press, 1985.

81   Freud, Sigmund. *The Future of an Illusion.* New York: W. W. Norton and Company, 1989.

81   _____. *Totem and Taboo.* New York, London: W. W. Norton and Company, 1989.

82   Hayman, Ronald. *A Life of Jung.* New York, London: W. W. Norton and Company, 1999.

82   Harding, Ester. The "I" and the "Not-I". *A Study in the Development of Consciousness.* Princeton, New Jersey: Princeton University Press, 1993.

82-83 Jung, C. G. *Psychological Types.* "Psychological Aspects of the Mother Archetype". p. 79 Princeton: Princeton University Press, 1971

83   Reik, Theodor. *The Search Within.* New York: Minerva Press, 1956.

83   Neumann, Erich. *The Origins and History of Consciousness.* Princeton: Princeton University Press, 1973.

83   Berne, Eric. *Transactional Analysis in Psychotherapy.* New York: Grove Press Inc., 1961.

83   Cobb, S. "On the Nature and Locus of Mind." *Archives of Neurology and Psychiatry* 67, 1952. p. 172-177.

84   Berne, Eric. ibid.

CHAPTER 6: FLESH APPEARS ON THE MIND

87   Klinger, Eric. *The Structure and Function of Fantasy.* New York: Wiley-Interscience, 1971. p. 107

87   ibid. p. 113

87   Ingles, Brian. *A History of Medicine.* Cleveland, Ohio: The World Publishing Company, 1965.

88   Porter, R. *The Greatest Benefit to Mankind: A Medical History of Humanity from Antiquity to the Present.* New York: Harper Collins, 1997.

88-89 Ploog, D. W. and MacLean P.D. "Display of Penile Erection in Squirrel Monkeys." *Animal Behavior.* 1963. p. 32-39.

89   Damasio, Antonio R. *Descartes' Error.* New York: Avon Books, 1994.

90   McCain, Alyson and Gordon, Stewart M.D. "What PET Scans of Neglected and Abused Children Reveal." *Seattle Times.* September, 2006.

90   Wilbur, Ken. *Up From Eden.* Boulder, Colorado: Shambhala Press, 1983.

PART III: HOW AN INDIVIDUAL HUMAN RECAPITULATES HUMAN EVOLUTION.

118   Shepherd, Gordon. *Neurobiology*. London: Oxford University Press, 1994.

118-119 Harris, Harold, editor. *Astride the Two Cultures, Arthur Koestler at 70*. re: Paul D. MacLean. New York: Random House 1976.

118-119 MacLean, Paul D. "The Brain's Generation Gap: Some human Implications." *Journal of Religion and Science*. USA: Zygon, Vol. 8 No. 2, June 1973.

120   Berne, Eric, MD. *Games People Play*. New York: Random House, 1967.

120   Horney, Karen. *Our Inner Conflicts*. New York: Norton, 1945.

122   Darwin, Charles. *The Expression of the Emotions in Man and Animals*. New York: New York Philosophical Library, 1872.

124   Tinbergen, M. *The Study of Instinct*. Oxford: The Clarendon Press, 1951.

124   Erickson, Mark T. Chapter 9: "Evolutionary Thought and Clinical Understanding of Incest." from *Inbreeding, Incest, and the Incest Taboo*. Wolf, Arthur P. and Durham, William H. editors. Stanford, California: Stanford University Press, 2005.

125   *Webster's New World Dictionary of the American Language*. Guralnik, David B., Editor in Chief, New York: William Collins + World Publishing Co., 1976.

126   Fromm, Erich. *The Anatomy of Human Destructiveness*. New York: Henry Holt and Co., 1973.

132   Laing, R. D. and Esterson, A. *Sanity, Madness and the Family*. London: Penguin Books, 1964.

CHAPTER 4: THE SIMIAN ELEMENT OF SELF

134   Bulfinch, Thomas. ibid.

135-136 MacLean, Paul D. *The Triune Brain in Evolution: Role in Paleocerebral Functions*. New York: Plenum Press, 1990.

135-136 Wright, Karen. "The Tarzan Syndrome." *Discover* November, 1996.

136   Howe, Mark. "An Infant's First Sense of Self" *Developmental Review* 23 (2003).

138   Laing, R. D. *The Politics of the Family and Other Essays*. New York: Pantheon Books, 1969.

CHAPTER 5: THE HOMINID ONTOGENY OF
    THE HUMAN SENSE OF SELF

145   Todd, James T., and Morris, Edward K. *Modern Perspectives on John B. Watson and Classical Behaviorism*. Connecticut: Greenwood Press, 1994.

145   Pavlov, Ivan. ibid.

146   Levy-Bruhl, Lucien. *The Soul of the Primitive*. translated by Clare, Lilian A. New York: The MacMillan Company, 1928.

149   Jaynes, Julian. ibid.

149   Mahler, S., Pine, M. M. and F., and Bergman, A. *The Psychological Birth of the Human Infant*. New York: Basic Books, 1973.

150   Rice, Edward. *Captain Sir Richard Francis Burton*. New York: Charles Scribner Sons, 1990.

151-152 Rutherfurd, Edward. *Sarum*. New York: Crown Publishers, Inc., 1987.

152   Rice, Edward. ibid. (quote) pages 111-112.

153   Jung, C. G. *The Psychology of the Unconscious: A Study of Transformations and Symbols of the Libido* Trans. Beatrice Hinkle. London: W. W. Norton and Company, 1916.

153-154 Wilson, Colin. *The Essential Colin Wilson*. Berkeley, California: Celestial Arts, 1986.

155   Horgan, John. "Mind Over Body: Stroke Victims Cannot Perceive Paralysis in Themselves or Others." *Scientific American*. September, 1996.

155   Rosenbek, John C. etal. "Effects of Two Treatments for Aprosodia Secondary to Acquired Brain Injury." *Journal of Rehabilitation Research & Development*. Vol. 43 No. 3 May/June 2006.

155   Macintyre, Ben. "Go to Work on an Ego: Why Spies Need the Last Word." www.timesonline.co. December, 2006.

156-157 Wilson, Colin. *Poltergeist*. London: Nel Books, 1981.

158   Laing, R.D. *The Divided Self.* New York: Pantheon Books, 1960

CHAPTER 6: VERTICAL INTEGRATION OF HUMAN SELF-IDENTITY

160   Shepherd, Gordon. *Neurobiology*. London: Oxford University Press, 1994.

161   Kappers, C. U. Ariens, Huber, G. Carl, and Crosby, Elizabeth Caroline. *The Comparative Anatomy of the Nervous System of Vertebrates Including Man*. New York: MacMillan, 1936.

162   Taylor, Gordon Rattray. *The Natural History of the Mind*. New York: E. P. Dutton, 1979.

163   Alexander, F. and Selesnick, S. *The History of Psychiatry*. New York: Harper and Row, 1966.

163   Duke-elder, Stewart. *System of Ophthalmology, The Eye in Evolution*. London: C.V. Mosby Company, 1958.

163   MacLean, Paul D. "The Evolution of Three Mentalities." *Man-Environment Systems* Vol. 5, No. 4. 1975.

166   Shepherd, Gordon. Ibid. re: Charles Bell and Francois Magendie.

169-170 Freeman, Walter J. *How Brains Make Up Their Minds*. New York: Columbia University Press, 2001.

171   Lee, John R., M.D. "The Triune Brain." *Somatics*. Spring, 1980. pp. 17-20

176   Laing, R.D. *The Politics of the Family and Other Essays*. New York: Pantheon Books, 1969.

176   Reik, Theodor. *The Search Within*. New York: Minerva Press, 1956.

176   Berne, Eric. *Transactional Analysis in Psychotherapy*. New York: Grove Press, Inc., 1961

177   Ranson, Stephen and Clark, Sam. *Anatomy of the Nervous System*. Philadelphia: B. W. Saunders Company, 1953. re: Broca.

179   Mac Lean, Paul D. *The Triune Brain in Evolution: Role in Paleocerebral Functions*. New York: Plenum Press, 1990.

180   Bard, P. "A Diencephalic Mechanism for the Expression of Rage with Special Reference to the Sympathetic Nervous System." *Amer. J. Physiol.* 1928, 844; 490-513.

180-181 MacLean, Paul D. Ibid.

182 *Merriam-Webster's Medical Desk Dictionary.* Springfield, Massachusetts: Merriam-Webster, Inc, 2005. re: Jacobson's organ.

184-185 Shepherd, Gordon. Ibid. re: John Hughlings Jackson.

184-185 Delacato, Carl H. *The Diagnosis and Treatment of Speech and Reading Problems.* Springfield, Illinois: Chas. Thomas, 1964.

184-185 Finger, Stanley. *Origins of Neuroscience: A History of Explorations into Brain Function.* U.S.: Oxford University Press, 1994. re: Phillip Bard and Walter Cannon

CHAPTER 7: HORIZONTAL INTEGRATION OF THE
HUMAN SELF-IDENTITY COMPONENTS

189 Weinburger, Eliot, editor. *Selected Non-Fiction Jorge Luis Borges.* New York: Penguin Books, 1999.

190 Haldane, E. S. and Ross, G. R. T. *The Philosophical Works of Descartes.* Cambridge Mass: The Cambridge University Press, 1967.

191 Stevenson, Robert Louis. *The Strange Case of Dr. Jekyll and Mr. Hyde and Other Stories.* ed. Jenni Calder. Harmondsworth: Penguin Books, 1979.

191-192 MacLean, Paul D. "The Evolution of Three Mentalities." *Man-Environment Systems* vol. 5, no. 4, 1975.

195-196 Duke-elder, Stewart. *System of Ophthalmology, The Eye in Evolution.* London: C, V. Mosby Co., 1958.

198 Poldrack, Russell A. and Packard, Mark G. "Competition Among Multiple Memory Systems: Converging Evidence From Animal and Human Brain Studies" *Neuropsychologia.* vol. 41, no. 3, 2003. pp. 245-251.

200 Springer, S. P. and Deutsch, G. *Left Brain, Right Brain.* San Francisco: W. H. Freeman and Company, 1981.

200 Laing, R. D. *The Divided Self.* New York: Pantheon Books, 1960.

201 Gardiner, H. *The Shattered Mind.* New York: Knoph, 1975.

201 Bandler, Richard and Grinder, John. "Patterns of the Hypnotic Techniques of Milton H. Erickson, M.D." *Meta Publications.* vol. 1, 1975.

201-202 Wilson, Colin. *The Essential Colin Wilson.* Berkeley, California: Celestial Arts, 1986.

202 Greenspan, Stanley I. and Shanker, Stuart G. *The First Idea.* Cambridge, Massachusetts: De Capo Press, 2004.

204 Wellman, K. *La Mettrie. Medicine, Philosophy and Enlightenment.* Durham: Duke University Press, 1992.

204-205 Penfield, Wilder. "Memory Mechanisms" *Archive of Neurology and Psychiatry* 67, 1952. pp. 178-198.

204-208 Penfield, Wilder. *The Mystery of the Mind.* Princeton, New Jersey: Princeton University Press, 1978.

206 Freeman, Walter J. *How Brains Make Up Their Minds.* New York: Columbia University Press, 2001.

210   Jaynes, Julian. ibid.

211   Pais, Abraham. *Subtle is the Lord: The Science and the Life of Albert Einstein*. New York: Oxford University Press, 2005

211-212 Springer, S. P. and Deutsch, G. *Left Brain, Right Brain*. San Francisco: W. H. Freeman and Company, 1981.

213   Orhnstein, R. *The Nature of Human Consciousness*. San Francisco: W. H. Freeman, 1987.

214-215 Eccles, J. C. and Gibson, W. C. *Sherrington: His Life and Thought*. Berlin: Springer-Verlag, 1979.

216   Restak, Richard. ibid. re: Broca and Wernicke

218   Laing, R. D. *The Divided Self.* New York: Pantheon Books, 1960.

218-291 Haley, Jay. *Strategies of Psychotherapy.* New York: Allyn & Bacon, 1963

CHAPTER 8: ADULT HUMAN ONTOGENY

223-234 Huxley, Francis. *Affable Savages: An Anthropologist Among the Urubu Indians of Brazil*. London: Hart-Davis, 1963.

224   Hutschnecker, Arnold A., M.D. *The Will to Live*. New York: Cornerstone Library, 1977.

224   Alexander, F., M.D. and Selesnick, S., M.D. ibid.

224   Holmes, Thomas, M.D. "Life Situations, Emotions and Disease." *Psychosomatics*. 19, 1978. pp. 747-54.

224-226 Horne, Michael H., M. D. "Object Relations: Theory and Practice." Grand Rounds of Psychiatry and Behavioral Sciences at the University of Washington School of Medicine, April 12, 2006.

226   Horne, Michael H., M.D. ibid.

226   Ader Robert, Felton, David L. and Cohen, Nicholas. ibid.

226   Sapolsky, Robert, M.D. "Stress and Health: From Molecules to Societies" Georgia State University, December 2005.

228   Manchester, William. *American Caesar: Douglas MacArthur 1880-1964*. New York: Dell Publishing, 1978.

228-229 R4 Residents' Presentation "The Truth about Lemmings: A Discussion on Group Process" Grand Rounds Psychiatry and Behavioral Sciences. University of Washington School of Medicine. March 30, 2006.

230-231 Dworetzky, Murray M.D. and Cohen, Sheldon M.D. (editors) "Portier, Richet and the Discovery of Anaphylaxis: A Centennial." *Journal of Allergy and Clinical Immunology* Vol. 110 #2 August, 2002.

231   Matzinger, Polly "The End of Self" *Discover Magazine*. April, 1996.

231-232 Livingstone, David *Last Journals of David Livingstone in Central Africa* USA: Dodo Press, 2003

CHAPTER 9: THE SENSE OF SELF AND MIND-BODY DISEASES

234-235 Ader, Robert, Felton, David L. and Cohen, Nicholas. ibid.

236-237 Sigal, Leonard H. and Yacov, Ron. ibid.

240   Brain, Russell. Diseases of the Nervous System. London: Oxford Press, 1956.

EPILOG

224   Greenspan, Stanley I. and Shanker, Stuart G. ibid.

Bibliography

Ader, Robert. Felton, David L. and Cohen, Nicholas. *Psychoneuroimmunology*. 4th edition New York: Academic Press, 2006.

Alberti, Robert E. and Emmons, Michael. *Your Perfect Right*. San Luis Obispo, CA.: Impact Publishers, 1986.

Akugustinac, Jean et. al. "Detection of Entorhinal Layers Using Tesla Magnetic Resonance Imaging" *Annal of Neurology*. 2005.

Alexander, F., M.D. and Selesnick, S., M.D. *The History of Psychiatry*. New York: Harper and Row, 1966.

Altholz, Josef L. "The Huxley-Wilberforce Debate Revisited." *Journal of the History of Medicine and Allied Sciences*. No. 35 (1980) 313-316.

Aries, Philippe and Duby, Georges, general editors. *A History of Private Life*. Cambridge, Massachusetts: Belknap Press, 1989.

"Baboons, Humans and Stress, the Cost of Being an SOB" *Yale Medicine*. Winter 2007.

Bandler, Richard and Grinder, John. "Patterns of the Hypnotic Techniques of Milton H. Erickson, M.D." vol. 1 *Meta Publications*. 1975.

Berne, Eric, M.D. *Games People Play*. New York: Random House, 1967.

_____ *The Structure and Dynamics of Organizations and Groups*. New York: Grove Press Inc., 1963.

_____ *Transactional Analysis in Psychotherapy*. New York: Grove Press, Inc., 1961.

Bloom, Benjamin S. *All Our Children Learning*. New York: McGraw Hill, 1980.

Boyd, William. *Textbook in Pathology*. Philadelphia: Lea and Febiger, 1953.

Bradbury, Ray. *The Stories of Ray Bradbury*. New York: Knopf, 1980.

Brain, Russell. *Diseases of the Nervous System*. London: Oxford Press, 1956.

Brash, J.C. and Jamieson, E. B. *Cunningham's Textbook of Anatomy*. London: Oxford University Press, 1974.

Brena, Steven F. *Yoga and Medicine*. Baltimore: Penguin Books, 1973.

Brentano, Franz. *Descriptive Psychology*. transl. by Benito Muller, London: Routledge, 1982

Brumberg, Joan. *The Body Project*. New York: Random House, 1997.

Buchbaum, Ralph. *Animals Without Backbones*. Chicago: Chicago Press 1948.

Bulfinch, Thomas. *The Age of Mythology*. Boston: S.W. Tilton and Co., 1894.

Campbell, Joseph. "Myths To Live By" *Bill Moyers Journal.* 1981.

Cobb, S. "On the Nature and Locus of Mind." *Archives of Neurology and Psychiatry.* vol. 67, 1952.

Coleman, James C. *Abnormal Psychology and Modern Life.* Chicago: Scott Foresman and Co., 1984.

Collins, Treacher F. *Arboreal Life and the Evolution of the Human Eye.* Philadelphia: Lea and Febiger, 1922.

Columbia Encyclopedia. New York: Columbia University Press, 1963.

Crosby, Harry. *The Cave Painting of Baja California.* San Diego, Calif.: Sun Belt Publication, 1997.

Damasio, Antonio R. *Descartes Error.* New York: Avon Books, 1994.

Darwin, Charles. *The Expression of the Emotions in Man and Animals.* New York: New York Philosophical Library, 1872.

———————. *The Origin of the Species.* New York: Random House, 1979.

Davis, Michael, PhD. "The Role of NMDA Receptors in Extinction of Fear" Grand Rounds Presentation, Department of Psychiatry and Behavioral Sciences, University of Washington, May 11, 2006. de Camp, L. Sprague. *The Great Monkey Trial.* New York: Doubleday, 1968.

Delacato, Carl H. *The Diagnosis and Treatment of Speech and Reading Problems.* Springfield, Ill.: Chas Thomas, 1964.

Descartes, Rene. *Passions of the Soul.* Indiana: Hackett Publishing Co., 1989.

Diamond, Jared. *Guns, Germs and Steel: The Fates of Human Societies.* New York: W.W. Norton, 1997.

Diamond, S. *The Double Brain.* London: Churchill Livingstone, 1972.

"A Diencephalic Mechanism for the Expression of Rage With Special Reference to the Sympathetic Nervous System" *American Journal of Physiology.* 844, 1928.

Dubos, Rene Jules. *Pasteur and Modern Science.* New York: Anchor Books, 1960.

Duke-elder, Stewart. *System of Ophthalmology, The Eye in Evolution.* London: C.V. Mosby Co., 1958.

Durrell, Lawrence. *Caesar's Vast Ghost.* New York: Arcade Publishing, 1990.

Dusheck, Jennie. "The Interpretation of Genes" *Natural History.* vol. 6, October, 2002.

Dworetzky, Murray, M.D. and Cohen, Sheldon, M.D. editors. "Portier, Richet, and the Discovery of Anaphylaxis: A Centennial" *Journal of Allergy and Clinical Immunology.* Vol. 110 #2 August, 2002.

Eccles, J.C. and Gibson, W. C. *Sherrington: His Life and Thought.* Berlin: Springer-Verlag, 1979.

"Erickson, Mark T. "Evolutionary Thought and Clinical Understanding of Incest" Chapter 9 from *Inbreeding, Incest and the Incest Taboo.* Wolf, Arthur P. and Durham, William H. editors. Stanford, California: Stanford University Press, 2005.

Finger, Stanley. *Origins of Neuroscience: A History of Explorations into Brain Function.* U.S.: Oxford University Press, 1994.

Foch, Ferdinand. *The Principles of War.* London: Chapman and Hall, 1921.

Foucault, Michel. "Freudian Superego Power." *Civilization.* January-February, 1996.

Freeman, Walter J. How Brains Make Up Their Minds. New York: Columbia University Press, 2001.

Freud, Sigmund. Civilization and Its Discontents. New York: W. W. Norton and Company, 1989.

————————. Collected Papers. New York: Basic Books, Inc., 1959.

————————. Dictionary of Psychoanalysis. Greenwich, Connecticut: Fawcett Publications, 1958.

————————. The Future of an Illusion. New York: W. W. Norton and Company, 1989.

————————. A General Introduction to Psychoanalysis. Liveright Publishing Corporation, 1924.

————————. Totem and Taboo. New York: W. W. Norton and Company, 1989.

Frishberg, Manny. "A Seattle Institute Picks Up Where the Genome Project Left Off." Seattle Metropolitan. July, 2006.

Fromm, Erich. The Anatomy of Human Destructiveness. New York: Henry Holt and Company, 1973.

Galin, David. "Implications for Psychiatry of Left and Right Cerebral Specialization." Archives of General Psychiatry. 1974.

Gardiner, H. The Shattered Mind. New York: Knoph, 1975.

Gazzaniga, Michael S., Le Doux, Joseph E. and Wilson, David H. "A Divided Mind." Annals of Neurology 2, 1977: 417-421.

Goetz, C. G., Bonduelle, M. and Gelfand, T. Charcot: Constructing Neurology. New York: Oxford University Press, 1995.

Gooch, Stan. Total Man. New York: Ballantine Books, 1974.

Greenspan, Stanley I. and Shanker, Stuart G. The First Idea. Cambridge, Mass.: DeCapo Press, 2004.

Haines, Duane E. Fundamental Neuroscience, 2nd Edition. Philadelphia: Churchill Livingston, 2002.

Haldane, E. S. and Ross, G. R. T. The Philosophical Works of Descartes. Cambridge, Mass: The Cambridge University Press, 1967.

Haley, Jay. Strategies of Psychotherapy. New York: Grune and Straton, Inc. 1963.

Harding, Ester. The "I" and the "Not-I". A Study in the Development of Consciousness. Princeton, New Jersey: Princeton University Press, 1993.

Harris, Harold, editor. Astride the Two Cultures. Arthur Koestler at 70. New York: Random House, 1976.

Harrison, T. R. Principles of Internal Medicine. New York: The Blakiston Company, 1950.

Hayman, Ronald. A Life of Jung. New York, London: W. W. Norton and Company, 1999.

Hebb, D. O. The Organization of Behavior. New York: Wiley, 1949.

Henig, Robin Marantz. Monk in the Garden: The Lost and Found Genius of Gregor Mendel, the Father of Genetics. Boston: Houghton Mifflin, 2000.

Hinde, R. A. Non-Verbal Communication. Cambridge, Mass: The University Press, 1972.

Hofstadter, Douglas R. and Dennett, Daniel C. editors. The Mind's "I". New York, Toronto: Bantam Books, 1982.

Holmes, Thomas, M.D. "Life Situations, Emotions, and Disease." Psychosomatics. No. 19. 1978.

Horgan, John. "Mind Over Body: Stroke Victims Cannot Perceive Paralysis in Themselves or Others." *Scientific American.* September, 1996.

Horne, Michael H., M.D. "Object Relations: Theory and Practice." Grand Rounds of Psychiatry and Behavioral Sciences at the University of Washington School of Medicine, April 12, 2006.

Horney, Karen. *Our Inner Conflicts.* New York: Norton, 1945.

Howe, Mark, Courage, Mary L. and Edison, Shannon C. "When Autobiographical Memory Begins" *Developmental Review.* No. 23, 2003.

Hutschnecker, Arnold A., M.D. *The Will To Live.* New York: Cornerstone Library, 1977.

Huxley, Francis. *Affable Savages: An Anthropologist Among the Urubu Indians of Brazil.* London: Hart-Davis, 1963.

Idriess, Ian L. *Our Living Stone Age.* Melbourne, Australia: Angus and Robertson, 1963.

_____. *Our Stone Age Mystery.* Melbourne, Australia: Angus and Robertson, 1964.

Ingles, Brian. *A History of Medicine.* Cleveland, Ohio: The World Publishing Co., 1965.

Jaynes, Julian. *The Origin of Consciousness in the Break-Down of the Bicameral Mind.* Boston, Mass: Houghton Mifflin Company, 1976.

Jung, C. G. *Psychological Types.* Princeton, New Jersey: Princeton University Press, 1971.

_____ *Psychology of the Unconscious: A Study of Transformations and Symbols of the Libido.* Trans. Beatrice Hinkle. London: W. W. Norton and Company, 1916.

Kappers, Ariens C.U., Huber, G. Carl, Crosby, Elizabeth Caroline. *The Comparative Anatomy of the Nervous System of Vertebrates Including Man.* New York: MacMillan, 1936.

Kaye, Robert, Oski, Frank, Barness, Lewis. *Core Textbook of Pediatrics.* Philadelphia: J, B. Lippincott Co., 1978.

Kin, Warren. "U. W. Researcher Ties Autism to Face-Recognition Trouble." *Seattle Times.* Wednesday, April 18, 2001.

Klinger, Eric. *The Structure and Function of Fantasy.* New York: Wiley Interscience, 1971.

Korzybski, Alfred. *Science and Sanity.* Lakeville, Connecticut: The International Aristotelian Library, 1958.

Kraepelin, Emil. *Psychiatry: A Textbook for Students and Physicians.* USA: Science History Publications, 1990.

Kramer, Samuel Noah. *From the Tablets of Summer.* Colorado: Falcon Wing Press, 1956.

Laing, R. D. *The Divided Self.* New York: Pantheon Books, 1960.

_____ *The Politics of the Family and Other Essays.* New York: Pantheon Books, 1969.

Laing, R. D. and Esterson, A. *Sanity, Madness and the Family.* London: Penguin Books, 1964.

LeDoux, Joseph. *The Emotional Brain: The Mysterious Underpinnings of Emotional Life.* New York: Touchstone, 1998.

Lee, John R. "The Triune Brain." *Somatics.* Spring, 1980.

Levy, J. *Psychobiological Implications of Bilateral Asymmetry. Hemisphere Function in the Human Brain.* Diamond, S. J. and Beaumont, J. G. editors. New York: John Wiley and Sons, 1974.

Levy-Bruhl, Lucien. *The Soul of the Primitive.* trans. Clare, Lilian A. New York: The MacMillan Company. 1928.

Livingstone, David. *Last Journals of David Livingstone in Central Africa.* New York: Harper and Brothers, 1875.

Lorenz, Konrad. *On Aggression*. New York: Harcourt, Brace and World, Inc., 1966.

MacIntyre, Ben. "Go to Work on an Ego: Why Spies Need the Last Word." www.timesonline. com. December, 2006.

MacLean, Paul D. "Brain Function and Socio-Sexual Behavior." *Contemporary Sexual Behavior Critical Issues in the 1970's.* Zubin, Joseph and Money, John editors. Baltimore: Johns Hopkins University Press, 1973.

_____ "The Brain's Generation Gap; Some Human Implications." *The Journal of Religion and Science.* Vol 8, No 2, June 1973.

_____ "The Evolution of Three Mentalities." *Man-Environment Systems.* Vol. 5, No 4 1975.

_____ "The Imitative Creative Interplay of Our Three Mentalities". *U.S. Department of Health, Education and Welfare.* 1975.

_____ "The Limbic System and Its Hippocampal Formation." *Neurosurgery* Vol. 2, 1954.

_____ *The Triune Brain in Evolution: Role in Paleocerebral Functions.* New York: Plenum Press, 1990.

Mahler, S., Pine, M.M., and F., and Bergman, A. *The Psychological Birth of the Human Infant.* New York: Basic Books, 1973.

Manchester, William. *American Caesar: Douglas MacArthur 1880-1964.* New York: Dell Publishing, 1978.

Manchester, William. *A World Lit Only By Fire.* Boston, Mass: Little, Brown and Co, 1993.

Matzinger, Polly. "The End of Self." *Discover Magazine.* April 1996.

"Mens Sana in Corpore Sano Editorial" *Annals of Internal Medicine* Vol. 144 No 2 January 2006.

Michener, James. *Hawaii.* New York: Random House, 1959.

Missenard, Andre. *In Search of Man.* New York: Hawthorne Books, 1957.

Morell, Virginia. "Kings of the Hill?" *National Geographic.* November 2002.

Netter, Frank H., M.D. "The Nervous System" *The Ciba Collection of Medical Illustration.* Vol. 1 New York: Ciba Pharmaceutical Company, 1979.

Neumann, Erich. *The Origins and History of Consciousness.* Princeton: Princeton University Press, 1973.

Nierenberg, G. L. and Calero, Henry H. *How to Read A Person Like a Book.* New York: Hawthorne Books, 1971.

Nin, Anais. *The Diary of Anais Nin 1931-1934.* New York: The Swallow Press, 1966.

O'Donnell, J. *The Origins of Behaviorism: American Psychology, 1870-1920.* New York: NYU Press, 1985.

Orhnstein, R. *The Nature of Human Consciousness.* San Francisco: W. H. Freeman, 1987.

Ouspensky, P. D. *The Psychology of Man's Possible Evolution.* New York: Vintage Books, 1974.

"Pain Fibers to the Brain" *Resident and Staff Physician.* December, 1983.

Pais, Abraham. *Subtle is the Lord: The Science and the Life of Albert Einstein.* New York: Oxford University Press, 2005.

Penfield, Wilder. "Memory Mechanisms" *Archive of Neurology and Psychiatry* 67, 1952.

——————— *The Mystery of the Mind*. Princeton, New Jersey: Princeton University Press, 1978.

Perry, et. al. "Retinal Arteriolar Occlusion in Multiple Sclerosis." *Annal of Ophthalmology*. 1986.

Ploog, D. W. and MacLean, P. D. "Display of Penile Erection in Squirrel Monkeys." *Animal Behavior.* 1963.

Porter, R. *The Greatest Benefit to Mankind: A Medical History of Humanity from Antiquity to the Present*. New York: Harper Collins, 1997.

Ranson, Stephen. Clark, Sam. *Anatomy of the Nervous System*. Philadelphia: B. W. Saunders Co., 1953.

Reik, Theodor. *The Search Within*. New York: Minerva Press, 1956.

Restak, Richard M., M.D. *The Brain*. Toronto: Bantam Books, 1984.

Rice, Edward. *Captain Sir Richard Francis Burton*. New York: Charles Scribner Sons, 1990.

Romer, Alfred Sherwood. *Man and the Vertebrates*. Chicago: University of Chicago Press, 1948.

Rosenbek, John C., et. al. "Effects of Two Treatments for Aprosodia Secondary to Acquired Brain Injury." *Journal of Rehabilitation Research and Development*. Vol 43 No 3 May/June 2006.

Rutherfurd, Edward. *Sarum*. New York: Crown Publishers, Inc., 1987.

Sagon, Carl. *The Dragons of Eden*. New York: Ballantine, 1997.

Sakai, Kuo and Nakana, Ide. *The Art of Lying*. New York: Red Brick Press, 1996.

Sapolsky, Robert, M.D. "Stress and Health: From Molecules to Societies". Georgia State University Presentation. December, 2005.

Scheie, H. G. and Albert, D. A. editors. *Textbook of Ophthalmology*. Philadelphia: W. B. Saunders Co., 1997.

Senet, Andre. *Man In Search of His Ancestors*. Boston: McGraw Hill Books, 1995.

Shastid, Thomas. *Our Own and Our Cousins' Eyes*. Southbridge, Mass: American Optical Company Publication, 1926.

Shepherd, Gordon. *Neurobiology*. London: Oxford University Press, 1994.

Sigal, Leonard H. and Yacov, Ron. *Immunology and Inflammation*. New York: McGraw Hill, Inc., 1994.

Sorenson, Roger W. M. D. "Clan Ego and Duo Ego." Unpublished papers and personal correspondence.

Spengler, Oswald. *The Decline of the West*. New York: A. Knoph, 1939.

Springer, S. P. and Deutsch, G. *Left Brain, Right Brain*. San Francisco: W. H. Freeman and Company, 1981.

Stenhouse, T. B. H. *The Rocky Mountain Saints*. New York: Appleton and Company, 1873.

Stevenson, Robert Louis. *The Strange Case of Dr. Jekyll and Mr. Hyde and Other Stories*. ed. Jenni Calder. Harmondsworth: Penguin Books, 1979.

Taguchi, Keiko et. al. "Identification of Hippocampus-Related Candidate Genes for Alzheimer's Disease." *Annals of Neurology*. 2005.

Taylor, Gordon Rattray. *The Natural History of the Mind*. New York: E. P. Dutton, 1979.

Teilhard de Chardin, Pierre. *The Phenomenon of Man*. New York: Harper Row, 1959.

Tinbergen, M. *The Study of Instinct*. Oxford: The Clarendon Press, 1951.

Todd, James T. and Morris, Edward K. *Modern Perspectives on John B. Watson and Classical Behaviorism*. Connecticut: Greenwood Press, 1994.

Toynbee, Arnold (Joseph). *A Study of History Volume I: Introduction; The Geneses of Civilization*. Oxford: Oxford University Press, 1934.

Uexkull, Jakob von. *Theoretical Biology*. New York: Harcourt, Brace and Co., 1926.

Weinburger, Eliot (editor). *Selected Non-Fiction Jorge Luis Borges*. New York: Penguin Books, 1999.

Wells, H. G. *The Outline of History*. New York: The MacMillan Company, 1921.

Wellman, K. *La Mettrie, Medicine, Philosophy and Enlightenment*. Durham: Duke University Press, 1992.

Wernicke, C. *Der Aphasische Symptomen Complex*. Breslau: Cohn and Weigert, 1874.

West-Eberhard, M. J. *Developmental Plasticity and Evolution*. New York: Oxford Press, 2003.

West, Willis. *The Ancient World*. Boston: Allyn and Bacon, 1913.

White, Ann Terry. *Men Before Adam*. New York: Random House, 1942.

Wilbur, Ken. *Up From Eden*. Boulder, Colorado: Shambhala Press, 1983.

Wilson, Colin. *The Essential Colin Wilson*. Berkeley, California: Celestial Arts, 1986.

_____. *Poltergeist*. London: Nel Books, 1981.

Wolf, Josef. *The Dawn of Man*. London: Thames and Hudson Publishing, 1978.

Worth, Claud. *Squint: Its Causes, Pathology and Treatment*. Philadelphia: Blakiston and Son Co., 1921.

Wright, Karen. "The Tarzan Syndrome" *Discover*. November, 1996.

Zubeck, John P. *Sensory Deprivation*. New York: Appleton-Croft, 1969.

www.ingramcontent.com/pod-product-compliance
Lightning Source LLC
Chambersburg PA
CBHW031827170526
45157CB00001B/217